Praise for *To Battersea Park*

'Beautiful … Works like this … allow the imagination to roam wide and wild'   *Observer*

'Powerful and propulsive … A book about the stories we tell ourselves about the pandemic; billions of stories, fragile, partial and essential, each one a small but vital act of reclamation and remembrance'   *Guardian*

'Magnificently succeeds in excavating the sedimentary layers of a neighbourhood in lockdown to reveal – hilariously, tenderly, shockingly – how we exist both in intimacy and ignorance of those we live among'   *Financial Times*

'Interesting and innovative … A different kind of state-of-the-nation novel; an exercise in imagination and empathy born out of a moment of collective crisis'   *Daily Telegraph*

'Eloquently distils the way in which enforced social distancing made us see the world around us through fresh eyes … Impressive'   *Mail on Sunday*

'Hensher is a gifted phrasemaker. He has the power to nail a character in an elegant line'   *The Times*

'Challenges everything we might have taught ourselves to expect from fiction … Ingenious'   *Times Literary Supplement*

'Richly strange ... A lockdown mosaic'   *Daily Mail*

'Playful, philosophical, sensual ... Above all, it's defiant: an account of confinement that refuses to be confined'
Literary Review

'One of our most consistently intelligent and beguiling writers'
WILLIAM BOYD, author of *The Romantic*

'The first great lockdown novel, and perhaps the only one we'll need'   MICK HERRON, author of *Bad Actors*

'An utterly engrossing skein of narratives, beautifully written and often disturbing'   LISSA EVANS, author of *V for Victory*

ALSO BY PHILIP HENSHER

FICTION
Other Lulus
Kitchen Venom
Pleasured
The Bedroom of the Mister's Wife
The Mulberry Empire
The Fit
The Northern Clemency
King of the Badgers
Scenes from Early Life
The Emperor Waltz
Tales of Persuasion
The Friendly Ones
A Small Revolution in Germany

NON-FICTION
The Missing Ink: The Lost Art of Handwriting

PHILIP HENSHER

TO BATTERSEA PARK

4th ESTATE • London

4th Estate
An imprint of HarperCollins*Publishers*
1 London Bridge Street
London SE1 9GF

www.4thEstate.co.uk

HarperCollins*Publishers*
Macken House, 39/40 Mayor Street Upper,
Dublin 1, D01 C9W8, Ireland

First published in Great Britain in 2023 by 4th Estate
This 4th Estate paperback edition published in 2024

1

Copyright © Philip Hensher 2023

A catalogue record for this book is
available from the British Library

ISBN 978-0-00-832314-1

Set in Adobe Garamond Pro
Printed and bound in the UK using 100%
renewable electricity at CPI Group (UK) Ltd

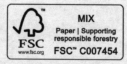

G.W.B.

All was done in love, anxiety, timidity,
stupidity and impatience.

SAMUEL BUTLER,
The Way of All Flesh

Errata: Page 320, for The fat one, *read* The fat ones.

ROBERT SMITH SURTEES,
Plain or Ringlets? (First edition, 1860)

CONTENTS

ONE

THE ITERATIVE MOOD

The State gave an order. We obeyed the order. Everyone obeyed the order. And the world changed.

For a long time I would get up early. Nothing was needed to wake me up. I would get out of bed, not waking my husband. I would leave the bedroom in my pyjamas, barefoot. I would close the door to the bedroom and its curtained dark, feeling the soft weight of the dressing-gowns and jackets swinging behind the door. I would take pleasure in the shift of sensation on the soles of my bare feet, from the coarse wool of the old Qashqai carpet in the bedroom to the hard wood on the landing. It always struck me as a change of texture and of temperature both. Other changes in texture and temperature followed as I walked through the house. If I went into the bathroom there would be the rippling sensation of tiles, and the once luxurious sensation of mechanical heat underfoot. Or in the rest of the house, more carpets, and a subtle shift from wood to what lay on the floor in the kitchen, an unrolled stretch of artificial stuff that I would once have confidently called *lino* and now seemed to have no name other than *floor covering*. The consideration of the name of the stuff on the floor in the kitchen was a regular one, and regularly called up the same train of thought, that if this stuff, once *lino*, was now called *floor covering*, then what was the wood in the rest of the house, not the house's pristine floorboards but a laid surface I had installed twenty years before? I felt that the names of things should preserve an obvious distinction. Almost every morning, after getting up between six and seven, I wondered whether this glacial blond surface was what used to be termed *parquet*, or whether that, too, had now been subsumed in the general term *floor covering*. I would come to no conclusion.

In all of this I would be obeying an order – the order of the State. The order concerned how, and for what reasons, we might leave our houses. The State decreed that we might not leave our houses for more than an hour a day. We were allowed to go outside for an hour's exercise, or to fetch essentials, but for no other reason. This was in March, when the surfaces of things carried the promise of infection and death, when the unfamiliar could not be touched, when strangers could not be allowed to approach closer than a coffin's length. We shut our doors. We stayed at home. We reflected on Engels' definition of the State as a 'special coercive force'. And time passed.

The house would be silent. The street outside would be silent. At most there might be the hushing sound of a broom over pavement, as Joe swept the empty pavements in front of his house, next to mine. That silence would not change as the day went on.

All through this time I would do the same things in the same order. I first made a sort of bread for breakfast. In the quiet kitchen, I would turn on the oven. I took down a greeny-brown package of buckwheat flour, mixing it with soda water and something to give it some flavour. I would take a dessertspoon and, with a forefinger, unload the glutinous wet dough, pocked with caraway seeds, onto a sheet of baking paper. I would resist the urge to lick my finger, driven by the memory of mixing cake batter when I was a child in my grandmother's kitchen; this grey gleaming dough held no secret appeal when raw, and not much when cooked. But it was good for you.

I would put the dollops of buckwheat mix into the oven, and make coffee. The automatic processes of the machine were thrilling to me, and their inconsiderate noises I always felt would wake my husband: the rattle of the beans falling into the reservoir and the shriek of the grinding mechanism. The machine had been in the kitchen for some years; it was only at this time, when the State had given an order and we obeyed the order, staying at home, that I had wondered what the term was for the part of the machine that the coffee fell into, that you pushed and twisted into a tight seal and let the boiling water drip through. I had looked at it daily, and wondered what the name for it was for some time, feeling at first that the name was obvious and it had only slipped my mind, before giving up and investigating. The part of the machine had a name: it was called a *portafilter*; I recoiled from the name with disappointment and scepticism. I would never use the word, even in my thoughts.

I pushed the handled *thing* forward, twisted and locked it, pressed a button, and the coffee dripped into the mug that was already there.

Things around me had acquired names in this time, names not subjective or based in my history or habits of use but ones with their own impregnable dignity and separation. *That carpet in the bedroom, the one I bought when I was twenty-one* was a sentence that had left me, like a child leaving home, and the carpet was now what it had always been, a Qashqai prayer mat, with so many knots per inch, with dyes of particular vegetables. I had turned back a corner of the carpet, like a favourite page in a novel, one quiet hour; I had counted the knots. The learning of names would be so slow, all through this period, and with so doubtful an outcome. The prayer carpet was as impregnated with ideas as its knots were with the red dye of madder root; it pointed backwards to my rewarding myself for getting my degree, carrying the mystery and the idea, too, of the price I could not understand how I could have paid, of £650 in 1986; it pointed still further backwards to its world of devotion, where God would be found in a particular direction, and the carpet would be oriented to aid the worshipper. It was saturated in meaning, and dripped, and the names I learnt were the guide to those once empty significances.

But not every name that had emerged had this meaning, or possessed any idea to enhance that raw physical substance. Sometimes it was just a name. At most it was a history. The *thing* that the coffee machine ground beans into was a *portafilter*; that was no name but a corporate label for a device, and the object's reality had been lost. I wouldn't use the word *portafilter* explaining the machine's processes to someone unfamiliar with them. I would say, *You push the sort of filter-holding thing into the slot underneath the kind of grinder*. But there was nobody to explain the processes to. My husband, who would still be in bed, had chosen not to learn how to use the machine, preferring that I would always make coffee for him. And there was nobody who might come into the house, except medical professionals. They, alone among strangers, would be permitted to enter; they would not make coffee. The name, once learnt and recoiled from with a little distaste, sat there, unused.

The machine did its work; the coffee was made. I would take the mug, one of six bought from a Charles Rennie Mackintosh museum, unimaginably far away in Glasgow and long ago, and open the back door into the garden. I would go out barefoot most days. I relished the shift of sensation, another change from the cooler parquet in the back passage to the stone of the ground outside, gritty however well swept, and with a depth of cold after the night that nothing would quite shift, a depth of cold that under these first steps would always strike me as the same thing as wetness. Sometimes it actually was wetness; I liked to take my coffee outside, barefoot, even if it had rained, and even if it was still raining. That shift of sensation would be in the air, too, a shift as if of strength of pressure between the interior household world of kitchen, passageways, red-curtained rooms, heated and controlled like a circus tent, and the open unroofed world of the garden and what lay above and beyond. It had once been a world of possibilities that that door opened into, as if you could enter the oxygenated garden, go beyond its fences into the world itself. But now the garden represented all there was in the world outside. You could not go beyond it, or only as far as half an hour's walk would take you, and then the world would come to an end. You would get to the gates of Battersea Park, and find that the time had come to turn back. I would not cross the river that lay a mile to the north for many months. As if in compensation, the world we were limited to by decree of the State, this garden and the house we lived in, had grown in the mind, and nothing was too small to look at, to name or rename, to contemplate.

The garden was small, a tarred terrace. It was a London outside space of twenty square metres, and without any ground soil. When I first lived here, the fence was swamped every year with a sea of jasmine. It was rooted in a neighbour's garden, but grew like a weed over my fence and for three years flooded the air for May and June with that odour of jasmine, so like bananas, so pure and unresisted that it felt aimed. I tried to keep up; I bought a few pots of hydrangeas, of pink fuchsias. Then one year the jasmine died; I don't know why. It was rooted in soil somewhere I could not see, and a neighbour must have taken some action against it. The hydrangeas and the fuchsias died soon too, of neglect. For years the terrace was a repository of rubbish bags and dead plants, the occasional daffodil bulb making an uncared-for revival.

But I came from a family of gardeners, and finally, in middle age, the urge, however frail at first, would assert itself, like a shoot of beech-wood that will in the end crack paving stones and show what the fecund earth underneath can do. We had cleared the terrace, and placed plants in containers all around. Some at first had died, quite quickly, It might be possible to grow a fig tree in a pot. But we could not. The ones that died or even faintly struggled were immediately despatched, and the ones that coped were replicated. So the garden I would go out into, the possibility of breeze opening up the sky above it, the three dozen windows around it keeping their opinions to themselves, was an experienced one. I would go round the containers carefully, inspecting each one, sometimes with a pair of blades to trim or shape. The three roses were prone to fly, and could be sprayed; I always felt, too, a deep joy during the long season between the first buds of their blooms showing themselves and their bursting into fullness, like wind-filled blouses on a line, the cream, the crimson, the opulent flurry with which the yellow in bloom flavoured the air by the kitchen door. There was a climbing and indestructible jasmine, a new one, its leaves fading daily from its winter scarlet to the innocent yellow-green I always associated with the key of A major, and by that, one of three camellias, finishing its flower-ing just as the jasmine started to limber up. There was a foaming cascade of convolvulus, its white trumpets like a licensed version of the bindweed I always loved as a child, dreamt of a garden buried in it; the fall of flowers buried a single piece of rubbish I had placed in the garden, like a recol-lection of that childish desire, and an old desktop hard drive lay rotting underneath a high-coiffured flood of bleached flower bells. There were two olive trees, each facing the other, most years to my astonishment producing a few olives as if they were in Greece. I had never known what olive blossom looked like, either, until now – the tiny beaded buds, the foam, the white flowers a millimetre wide. The olives every year would draw a bold squirrel into the garden; it would lean forward and pull at one, gigantic in its little paws, gnawing at it, like a drunk Gulliver at a cocktail party in Brobdingnag. And at the back a wall of bamboo, growing like a wildfire. Most weeks from spring onwards I would need to thin the bamboo of dead or browning shoots, and it always responded with a fresh green shoot, growing so quickly you could almost watch it move. By June the highest blades would be nine feet tall. Once in another life, in Japan, I had heard the creak of bamboo growing another millimetre, disbelieving. One day, in this life, I hoped to hear my bamboo in the two man-length tubs creak joyously back.

There would be something new in the garden. There would be old things, too, which had lost their names soon after their installation, had somehow thrived. Those plants had discovered their own names again, since the State had forbidden us to go far from them. The tree that I had bought in the Sunday-morning market, with its brushlike vermilion flowers and cones like fingers, revealed itself to be a callistemon. A horticultural guest to lunch had once judged it to be *bedint*, an old Bloomsbury word for vulgar or common. I was amused. I loved the stately flourish of vermilion, a splash against the bamboo, the colour of an Inari gate, and no guest would come to put it in its place again, not for long concentrating months of excavation.

I would stand in the garden and relish what it held, the colours that had the licence to clash, reds against purple and white, cream against yellow. The variety of green leaf, too, I had begun to appreciate only through living with it, the verdant inner luminosity of the bamboo, like commercial supermarket salad, or the powdery greyish green, as elegant as sage, of the convolvulus leaves, or the camellia's villainous racing-green polish you could see your face in. Some days during this time I would come out and be struck by the smells, the perfume of the yellow roses by the door or the flowering jasmine or the bog myrtle's wash, like an expensive cologne, or just the smell of a garden after recent rain, the smell I now knew had been given a specific name within living memory. That new collision of rain and dry earth was called *petrichor*; it had always existed, that smell, and first been named in the 1960s. Petrichor. The name had caught on. I had just learnt it.

There was silence in the garden. The part of London I lived in was quiet, a back street lined with trees, but in those months you could almost reach out and squeeze the silence in the air, like a saturated sponge. Always before there had been the remote and steady grumble of traffic, like a sixty-four-foot organ stop played pianissimo in an empty cathedral; you felt it before you knew how to listen to it. And that was gone, like the exhaust particles that had stained the busy air. It was as if a headache had cleared, all at once. The sky would be empty, too, both of the planes, which in other times descended twice a minute towards the airport to the west, and, higher up, the planes that once had drawn slowly fattening lines in the deeper blue.

There was no silence, in reality. Even in the back garden, you could sometimes hear a faint slapping from the street as a neighbour set off on his or her daily permitted run. I heard these slaps of rubber on pavement, and liked to think of them joining a community of well-spaced runners in the park, where the mumbling clamour of footfall would fill the empty air, like the subdued and unending acclaim of a multitude. I would stand there and the animal sounds, the sounds as if of a forest, would make themselves felt: the hiss and warning roar of wind through the beech tree in the little recreation ground a hundred yards away. The burst of vermilion callistemon flowers and, by it, the high foxgloves with their imperial purple and white bell-flowers lined with blotches, they sent out a secret message on the air, and the muscular grumbling of bees started and stopped with purposeful abruptness. The lemon glisten of song from a blackbird, as if it knew that for once everyone was listening to the purity of its notes. Pigeons settled in trees, or perched on the top of chimneys, and made their indecisive but insistent *woo-woos* for hours on end. You could hear, too, the football rattle of an angry magpie, the shriek and clamour of those new Londoners, the jaunty savage mobs of parakeets. Everyone had a different explanation for how they had come to be here, driving out the flurrying sparrows of my London childhood, and nobody really knew.

I've never seen pigeons look so healthy, my husband had said one day. We had been standing at the front window. Outside a cherry tree was in bud. A London pigeon had been tugging at one bud after another, eating what it could. It looked slim, almost glossy with health, and yet somehow resentful, as pigeons do. We watched for a time.

Perhaps – I said – the London pigeon's usual diet has dried up. It's had to go back to eating what its ancestors ate, buds and insects.

What do you mean, the usual diet, my husband asked.

Discarded kebabs, I said. And the vomit of drunks on Clapham High Street. Sunday morning would be the best time. They must be discovering that it's not so good for them to eat everything from the pavement or rubbish bins.

A lesson worth learning, my husband said briskly, but we did not move from the front window. We would go on watching the pigeon try to eat the buds of the cherry tree, and after it flew off, we would watch the cherry tree in bud. It had recently stopped raining. The tree, wet, shone like a knife in the sun.

I would have finished my coffee. My bare feet would be cold, the chill spreading up my ankles. I would wait. There was no reason to go inside until the buckwheat rolls were baked. I had no idea what time it was and no nagging sensation that something had to be achieved, or perhaps just undertaken, at some point today. I would have a bath soon. My husband would get up; he liked to sleep longer than I did. And then the different tasks of the day would start, the same tasks every day, but undertaken cheerfully and with undisturbed, remote control. The life we lived was of the utmost habit, circling the day like a satellite, and in that habit resided a happiness I felt I had only glimpsed before. From one day to the next the only thing that changed were the clothes I wore and the novel, between breakfast and lunch, I would be reading. In the unquestioned following of habitual behaviour, like a spiritual exercise, I discovered happiness. During March I read nineteen novels by Ivy Compton-Burnett, one after the other, between breakfast at eight and lunch at one, starting a new one as soon as I had finished the last, like lighting each cigarette from the butt of the one before. During April I baked canelés bordelaises every afternoon, practising every day until they were quite perfect, glazed, hard-ridged, and producing an inside that was soft to the very edge of being liquid. After I had learnt to do them properly, I continued for a week, producing a perfect batch every afternoon. Then I stopped.

The practice of habit was that of a medieval peasant. Sometimes when we went out for a short walk before bedtime, I would be surprised if we did not see the silent, calculating fox of the neighbourhood sauntering down the middle of the road it now thought it owned. Our habits were more regular than those of a wild animal patrolling its narrow territory, and the source of deep undisturbed happiness. I was a writer; by inclination always; by profession for three decades. For the first time in my life I had not written a word for months.

The State had told us that we might go out once a day, for an hour, for the sake of exercise. We did so, and so did many of our neighbours. We got to know their habits and accustomed behaviour. Some of these other people were regular phenomena in the world that our small observations constructed. Joe next door swept the pavement before his house with a stiff witchy broom. He did this every day, though no rubbish could have accumulated; I thought it was a domestic habit he had inherited from his mother, who had learnt it from her mother in a chalky Calabrian street, where Joe himself had never been. Once in a while we heard him exchange a barbed and self-protective comment with the man who lived opposite, the nuisance. There was also a man who lived a few houses away we knew as the Jogger. In the morning we would see him in his exercise gear, loping past, his hands hanging down, his white-shod feet padding the pavements with a sombre unthinking rhythm. An hour later, we would see him return, his hair glistening, his face purple-dark and gasping, like a landed tropical fish. We would remark to each other that there the Jogger had gone. Each evening, with fresh exercise clothes, he ran out again, for a second hour, returning in the same condition. They were one of two Black families in the little street. The thoughtful mother and small, nervous, bookish son might not value their successful father's making a spectacle of himself; in any case they did not Jog.

We would take an hour's walk, strictly in accordance with the State's decree. It amused us, like an Uber driver deliberately irritating his passengers by sticking to the forty mile speed limit on the road from the airport. Always before, the few quiet streets around us had been a neutral zone with nothing much of interest to supply. We had passed through them quickly, still carrying the concerns of the house with us, or thinking about the place we were aimed for – Geneva, the London Library, a friend's lunch at his house in Belsize Park. Now an hour's walk restricted us to those few streets. We started to notice things.

If you turned right at the front door, and left again, you passed an Ethiopian church and were at the Queenstown Road. It was a road into and out of the centre of London; an *artery*, I had heard it called. On Monday mornings in normal times, the road would be static with traffic and metalled to a polished shine, as car against car waited for anything to change. If the traffic was like this and you needed to reach somewhere, it was best to walk for forty minutes, to cross the shining river by the shining fixed line of vehicles slashed across it, until you reached Chelsea. It was always busy. But now it was empty, unused, vacant. You could stand in the middle of the street and see nothing approaching from this side; turn and see nothing from the other. Once in this time, I lay down in the centre of the road, aligned with the useless road markings dividing the road in two. Supine, I remained there. It was noon. Nothing came on my right side, going towards Chelsea; nothing came on my left side, going towards Clapham. The sun was warm on my face and the silence was strong. After a time I lifted myself up. Quite near a vixen stood in the middle of the road, examining me with curiosity. She sauntered away and so did I.

I had walked down the Queenstown Road ten thousand times in these two decades without seeing anything much. There was nothing much to be seen. What I had seen were the couple of restaurants we had gone to and the shops we had used: the dry cleaners, the Argentinian steak house, the shop that had been an Oddbins and the Greek takeaway where a friend's boyfriend had worked, morose in his greeting behind the till when we waved from the street. Those were all shut; the friend's boyfriend had died. Now we saw more.

There was some fruit scattered and rotting in someone's front garden, behind a wall. This was newly unfamiliar. The Queenstown artery held kebab shops and takeaways, and in usual times the road was scattered with dropped food and detritus. But that was all gone now, and the scattered shopping in the little front garden had a freshly debauched air. Someone had emptied their grocery bags over the front wall of a block of mansion flats, and left everything there amid all the Queenstown tidiness. But there was something incomplete about the explanation that had come so quickly. I was getting better at understanding when you needed to look again, and I looked again. What I had thought was scattered grocery shopping was uniform, like the shopping of an obsessive starting a fad diet. What was scattered across the little yard were twenty or thirty fruits, yellow or touched with pink, each the size of a small child's head. We stood. I saw, underneath two grand trees, growing right against the walls and windows of the mansion block, scrabbling for earth in the eight feet of space between block and front wall. The trees were glossy and dark and unknown. I tipped my head back. There in the foliage dark were more fruit, hanging and glowing in the dense shadow like Chinese lanterns.

What is it, I said. I don't know what this tree is at all. They look like grapefruit.

Smell it, my husband said. He pulled a dark leaf from the twig and rubbed it between his fingers. He held his fingers to my face. His face was alive with pleasure. A flood of sharpness, and something like –

Is that … I said. It could be bergamot almost, I said.

Earl Grey, he said. You don't like Earl Grey. It's a pomelo. My grandfather had one in his garden in Dhaka.

A pomelo, I said, wondering.

Two pomeloes, he said. He was right. In this little space of earth, two thick-trunked trees grew. They were twenty-five feet high. When I tipped my head up and looked, the leaves met in a solid barrier, and the fruit shone in a green darkness that turned into deepest black. Do you think we could take some, my husband said.

I don't see why not, I said. They're just lying on the ground. Half of them are rotting. But be quick about it.

The door of the mansion block opened; somehow shyly, someone not wanting to be observed. A woman stood there, her hand on the doorknob, and smiling.

You like my trees, she said, very happily. You know what they are?

They look like pomeloes, my husband said.

Well done you, she said. Most people say grapefruit, big orange, or one lady, she said lemon. Lemon! Man from the Council, mind …

She trailed off, still smiling. Perhaps like other people she had not spoken to anyone else for some weeks now. She was neat, tiny, her bare arms bone and a sag of skin; in her high-boned yellowish face under a scribble of hair, the dark intelligent eyes shone like wet glass catching the light. Her face was not so much freckled as mottled, the face of a beauty brightly reflected in a salt-decayed mirror somewhere by a hot blue sea.

You want to take some pomelo? No problem, she said. I can't eat more than one each day. They going to stay there, rot, you take them, then. Nice to see you appreciate my trees. Come inside my garden, easier to gather. You want to see the trees from underneath? You'll value that sight, I can tell.

Her name was Marianne. The solitude had worn away at her in some ways. She was prepared and careful in her surfaces, her clothes clean and comfortable. She reminded me at once of those shy small beasts in Tove Jansson, the ones who live under a stove or beside a tree. They have forgotten their own names and have to be persuaded out, the ones out of whom words, in time, tumble. She talked about her trees, the big pomelo and the little one behind – these names were ancestral, clear in her mind. I could see no real difference in size between the two trunks. They were substantial trees. They were forty years old, the trees, Marianne said. Perhaps the big pomelo had grown faster than the little pomelo at some early stage of their lives, back in the 1980s.

I'm worried for the pomelo, one of the pomeloes I'm grow-ing, an imagined Marianne not thirty years old said, in my head.

They are doing just fine, a male voice said. Who was he? I could not think. A new man in Marianne's life, I thought, back in the 1980s. He was gone by now.

Yeah, the big pomelo, that is doing just fine, my imagined Marianne said. But the other one in the blue pot, the little one, I am not so confident over him. This week I am going to plant both of them in the soil, take them out of the pots, see which of them survives, but I am not hopeful for the little pomelo out of the two. That one struggling. And you need a lady pomelo and a gentleman pomelo for the fruit to come. My father, he told me. You need two. He was a civil servant, my father, very careful, very thoughtful, a man you want to take your advice from.

And then they were for ever the big pomelo and the little pomelo, those two trees. They were there, she now said to us, growing ten years or fifteen before they produced a first fruit. Before that, they had produced blossom in June and nothing followed. The blossom of the pomelo, Marianne said, is a beautiful thing. My father wrote in letters to me from Grenada that I would be happy to smell the blossom at least, close my eyes, and I'm in the pomelo orchard. He writes a beautiful letter, my father, and he's right. I told myself for years that I'm happy there's only blossom but no fruit. And I believe myself! But then fifteen years have gone by and for the first year there is one fruit growing on a branch. I cannot believe what I am seeing. I go out to see it every day. One day it is big enough to pick. And I fetch my stepladder that I have bought from the ironmonger's just there.

Do you know that ironmonger's over there? Marianne asked.

Yes, I said. It's a useful shop. They've got everything.

Him and his daughter! she said. Her and her Alsatian dog. Forty years I am going there and she don't say hello even, like she knows me. She is the one that laughs at me when I first say I am growing a pomelo tree. Little girl then behind her father's counter. A what, she says. The father comes out and goes back again, comes back with his dictionary. Who knows that man has a dictionary? That man thinks he knows everything. Looks in the big dictionary. Has to. Oh, a Po Me Low, he says.

Marianne reached up and scratched her head, pulled a disapproving downward face, like Stan Laurel. She was a good mimic once she got going, one who enjoyed herself and liked an audience. I knew that indispensable ironmonger, the old man and his unsmiling daughter with her gruff voice; their Alsatian did the smiling for both of them, teeth bared and chained in the window.

A Po Me Low, he says, said Marianne. That's what you can grow in where it is you come from. Well, you can't grow it here. Too cold, he says. Not wet enough. Get yourself a nice dahlia or two. They're nice if they aren't too brightly coloured. Where is it you come from, that's what he says. Not interested and he's going to pretend he's not remembered next time, so I

don't know why he's asking, so I don't know why I tell him.
Grenada, I say. Like the television company, he say. I do not
know what the poor foolish man is talking about. No, I say, it's
an island, and I buy the stepladder and leave it at that. I am
from Grenada, grew up there, been in this country forty years
now, a bit more. It's the pomeloes that have been here for all
those forty years. They grew all right. Doesn't matter what that
one says will grow or don't grow. They tell me I don't know but
I am right and it's them don't know. Look at my trees!

We looked up. The trees had the gloss and abundance of
pampered houseplants, drunk on Baby Bio. The fruit sang with
a preserved and transported light inside it. It might have been
placed there, like electrical decorations at Christmas, and not
be globes waiting to be taken away. Marianne had come from
Grenada a little more than forty years ago. Had we heard of
Grenada? We had. Had we been to Grenada? We had not. It
was beautiful. She did not want to leave it but she had had to
leave it. She had never been to London. She had heard of it.

Like you, Marianne said, heard of it, never gone visit it, you
with Grenada, me with London. She cackled, an ex-smoker's
dry cough; her teeth were big and only a little yellow with age.

In their garden in Grenada, there were eight pomelo trees.
An orchard. More fruit than anyone could eat. They gave the
fruit away to neighbours and friends of neighbours and a few
years let the man come and harvest them and sold them to
him. The time comes for Marianne to leave and go to this place
called London. She says to her father that she would like to
grow these trees in London. Her father had great respect for
the British. That was why she was going there, because of that
great respect. He always wanted to go there and would have
visited Marianne there. In the event he died in Grenada where
he was born, still talking about the visit he was going to make
to his daughter in London. Now, however, Marianne asked

him a question about the pomelo tree, and he looked very doubtful. The trees would not grow in London. It was too cold. You need good soil, too, for the pomelo. In London there must be metals and car fumes buried in the soil. He did not think it would be a success.

And also, her father said, it was perhaps a criminal thing to bring foreign plants into the United Kingdom that might be carrying all sorts of diseases. You did not want to start out on the wrong foot.

And all that might have been quite right, but Marianne said she did not want to go to London and take nothing with her. She was a stubborn girl. I have got much more laid back as I got older, Marianne said. I see the other person's point of view. I sometimes admit that they are right and I have been wrong. But that is only in recent times and I do not often admit anything of that sort. Then I was a stubborn girl.

Her father picked two fruit, one from this tree, one from that. Just in case, Marianne said. I saw him as Marianne talked. He was tiny, as she was, and sinewy, and pale-skinned and freckled, as she was; he darted up a ladder with frowning brisk-ness once, and then, the ladder under his arm, went to another tree, placing it against the trunk, testing it with a shake before dashing up again and taking another fruit. In the kitchen, he and Marianne sliced and chopped the flesh, taking one fruit each, and laid the seeds in a line on two sheets of foolscap paper. There were nine seeds from his fruit and eleven from hers. The next two days, the seeds on their sheets of paper lay on the windowsill in the sun, until they were dry. The two sheets of paper had been labelled.

This is an insurance policy, her father said. In case the cuttings fail. The day you leave, I will give you two cuttings, wrap them in wet cotton wool, see if they take. If not, the seeds.

When the time came and the seeds were ready, Marianne's father put one set of seeds in one envelope, the other in another. The two envelopes he had put a careful name on. This envelope was marked Seeds from the little tree, and this envelope Seeds from the big tree. So that she would know which shoots came from which tree and would be good to make a pollination happen, you understand?

I understood. Marianne's description of these two trees as the little pomelo and the big pomelo had nothing to do with their size now. They had been named from their parent trees by a man who would never see the children.

Take some of the fruit, Marianne said. There are too many for me. I like my neighbours more if they take them away. Within reason. I'll get you a couple of bags.

She was in and out in seconds, with crumpled orange plastic bags from Sainsbury's and two glasses of water that had not been offered or requested. I liked her gracious hospitality; we took the glasses and drank the South London tap water as it was offered, in a spirit of polite transaction. My husband bent and began to pick over the fallen pomeloes critically, taking the ones still whole and firm on the ground.

I always tell my father, mother about the trees when I write my letters home, Marianne said. They like to hear. One cutting takes and the other tree is from one of the seeds. Now they are the same. My father has the reputation of a good man for growing things, like he has some kind of magic touch. But the truth is that people are not interested in finding out the skill behind things. He is not a magician, my father, he is a civil servant, but God bless them for thinking otherwise, those people. They prefer to think there is just a magic touch, like somebody blessed or in the grip of some kind of inspiration, than to listen and find out that you can do this, do this, do this, best to plant here, use this kind of bone on this kind of earth. And then you do that, your tree will grow. My father, he's astonished in his letters to hear that the pomeloes are growing, one from the seed, one from the cutting he gave me. That is because when I am a girl at home in Grenada, I am not considered the gardener in my family. That is my sister Kathleen. Four children and nine grandchildren and never moved more than five miles from where she is born – it's a job to remember all their birthdays. I do it all by Moonpig these days, they deserve more than an email, I hope they know.

Marianne read her father's advice-filled letters carefully, and took them to the place she knew, the ironmonger's on the other side of the road, seventy yards away. Did she have a job? Or did she have children to look after? Like the new man in Marianne's life I had imagined, they were presences that could only be guessed at. They did not enter into her story. My husband went on turning the pomeloes over in a slow, almost enraptured way. Perhaps he was thinking of another pomelo tree, in his grandfather's garden; perhaps he knew the story would end when the supermarket bags had been filled.

The judging old man in the ironmonger's gave her what he could – perhaps bonemeal. He told her about the nursery that hunkered on the flanks of Wandsworth Prison a couple of miles away, and she went there by the 77 bus. They know me there by now, Marianne said, laughing. The old ones remember me because of coming in with a list of things and telling them they were needed to grow things. And asking them what the soil is round here, which is what my father said I had to know. They scratched their heads and said nobody ever, ever asked what the soil is in Wandsworth. Do you know what the soil is in Wandsworth? Very important when you want to grow anything in your garden.

I had no idea, and, still worse, had no idea that I could have had any idea. The ground in London was paved for me, and I had no concept that there was land beneath, or soil, except in the most general terms. I had a vague memory that the reason the Underground line skirted Battersea and went through Vauxhall to Clapham was that an ancient bog lay next to the river that the Victorians would not try to tunnel through. But that was all.

I wrote to my father, Marianne said, and told him what the soil is here, after they tell me. Nicholas who works at the nursery, he's a very knowledgeable scholar, the first kind man I ever met in England. We are friends forty years now. My father writes back airmail and he says, That soil will support your pomelo trees. And I am able to write back with Polaroid photographs saying that his advice is very welcome, but the information is too late. By the time the letter it arrives, the two pomelo shoots are in the ground and four feet, growing like nothing. They are very happy to be here. My father a little annoyed to hear that his advice was not needed. The next letter from my mother and all about my sister's new baby I recall, like he said, You write to your daughter, I cannot be troubled where my knowledge has no value. But it is all right in the end. The trees are doing very well, and they come through the winter with no fuss at all. Once I saw the man from the hardware or his daughter, grumpy old girl with her Alsatian, coming down the road towards my flat here and my garden with two trees in it, eight feet high by that time and full of untutored vigour, my father used to say when he approved of something. That girl she sees she is going to have to walk past the two trees that she knew would never grow in this country and she walks to the other side of the road with her Alsatian, looking in the other direction entirely. Growing ever since without a care in the world. After ten, fifteen years they start to give fruit. Never anything but joy from them. Just one bad thing happened, though. One day it was, twenty years ago now, the man from the Council ring on the door with his little clipboard and his little form and his little legal letter ... They look too big to you?

They looked wonderful, I said. They did. I had never seen anything like them, growing in a street in the middle of the city, clinging to the edge of soil that unexpectedly suited them, forty feet up rooted in eight feet of earth. Marianne's mood had changed with the memory of the man from the Council, whatever he had done, and her victory over the superior girl from the hardware shop. I knew the girl too; I could feel how sweet that victory might have been, and how it might nevertheless taint your joys with the reminder of yourself and how you had won. It was time for the small shy happy creature to go back inside, closing the door against the world she loved to look at. The memory of a patrolling heedless Groke had come to her, and had frozen the ground it sat on.

That was three dogs ago, mind you, Marianne said. She was still talking about the woman who worked at the hardware shop, her enemy. She's had another one and then another one, and now the one she has now. They are all called Sheba, like they are the same dog or something, one dies but it doesn't matter. Nice to meet you, nice you take the trouble to look in. Come back any time. Would be nice to see you again.

She wiped her hands on her apron, as if it had been her picking the pomeloes up off the floor, and her smile, which had been on without a break, brightened two or three degrees. Her hands twitched; she might have been about to offer to shake our hands. But she remembered her manners, the new ones the State required of us, and said goodbye with a little bend of the shoulders, a small shake of the head.

What happened with the Council? my husband asked, once we were home. We had been out for more than an hour, but less than an hour out of that had been exercise. We thought we could argue our case if it came to it. I didn't get that bit, he said.

I don't know, I said. Old foes, evidently. They can't stand it if they see something they haven't ordered to take place.

The man from the Council, my husband said fondly. I could see a comic character in the process of being born, a towering menace in gabardine and an ultramarine knitted tie.

We ate the first of the pomeloes in a salad with watercress, feta cheese and a heavy dusting of sumac; alongside a couple of slices of mackerel, it sang like birds in the trees. My manners had gone out of the window, and while eating my dinner I read on the computer in front of the place setting about the soils of Wandsworth. My husband sat on the sofa and ate; the thirteenth episode of the seventh series of a moronic American programme he was joyfully enduring unspooled in the background. Obese Americans were assuring each other that it was inner beauty that was important and that love was the glue, or perhaps cement, or perhaps bindweed, that glued or tied families together – I forget. The music swelled. In Wandsworth the soil was *Slowly permeable seasonally wet slightly acid but base-rich loamy and clayey soils*. The texture was *loamy and clayey*. With some delight I read that the soil was characteristic of *seasonally wet pastures and woodlands*. On the map, the soil formed a green ring around sand-coloured islands of acid, loamy territory of less fertility. We, and Marianne, had been lucky to live on *seasonally wet pastures and woodlands*. I read out the line to my husband, who murmured something noncommittal. I promised myself that the very next time I went out, I would see in my mind's eye those pastures and woodlands, pulsing under the brown- and red-brick terraces, the grey laid blanket of tarmacked roads, just waiting, like the sauntering fox on the Queenstown Road or Marianne's pomeloes, to take their opportunity and fill their acres. The land had always been there under the bus routes of South London, the hardware shops, the crack houses, the new-build opportunities, the Greek takeaways, the builders burrowing to create cellars under Victorian terraces, the Ethiopian churches and the unsuccessful steak restaurants, Marianne's house and mine, unseen pastures and lush, patient woodlands.

We lived between two parks, a common to the south, a park to the north. One had been wild land for centuries. It had been enclosed and defined for the city in the 1870s. The other was a sumptuous, encyclopaedic, landscaped park, with lakes, pagodas, winding paths, statuary and designed vistas. It had been made in the 1840s. They were our destination, in normal times, for walks. Now we could reach the gates of the park, perhaps venture in for a few minutes, and it was time to turn back again. In the body of the park the springtime mysteries were occurring: the waterbirds were nesting, and hatching their chicks, the goslings, the cygnets, the ducklings. Somewhere inside there the coots were making their swift piping arguments with each other; the swans were stretching their necks and hissing like hydrants at any threat to their children. The long promenade of cherry trees was bursting into its spring *hanami*, unvisited, unseen. The park was twenty minutes' walk away; near enough to reach; too far to enter. Both park and common were the destinations, too, for the Joggers that made themselves evident in these times, like the man who lived a few doors away, the man whose slapping tread we heard on the street every day. They could reach the park; but being Joggers, they saw nothing of it and would not notice when, as every year, one of the sharp-beaked herons ate half the clutch of cygnets, one by one, undeterred by the hiss and fury of the cygnets' parents.

The Jogger in our street. He, his wife and child were a family with a professional and serious aura, with a gleaming four-by-four outside – he had a fierce proprietorial approach to parking, his right to the three metres of space in front of his home. He was a lawyer or an administrator of some sort in the public service; his wife was a head teacher. But that role had been too much dwelt on. Nobody else had done what he had, built a new housing development, a shopping precinct, understood and exploited the laws of grants and planning to have created, from nothing, something that gleamed and shone and would stand for decades. Or perhaps he had succeeded only in closing down a takeaway restaurant with rat droppings under the sink. At the end the principles had produced what they were meant to. He and his wife were upstanding, honourable, and were admired, even loved, by hundreds of people who had passed under the transforming justice of their attention. He was baffled and bored by the expressions of that admiration, and perhaps by his own excellence – you felt that. Those principles had produced, in their son, a boy who loved to read above anything else, reading not for improvement but to discover who in these pages would be judged worthy of marrying the rich hero. The boy, in this city, at this time, had suffered for it and would suffer more. Before the end of this period of immuration his father would commit suicide.

And there were many of them, these Joggers. We tried, in the first days of the State's decree, to get to the park before our hour's permitted exercise began. We hoped for a quiet and undisturbed walk along the serpentine paths, that we would take in the modernist sculpture by the lake, the monument to the brown dog, victim of vivisection, the pagoda to the principles of peace. But it could not be done. Usually we reached the gates of the park, and turned back. The paths were taken up by the Joggers, perspiring and flailing, their faces irresolute and assured. It was inexplicable. The terror of other people had been drummed into us by the State's communications. We

understood that other people should not come within a coffin's
length of us, that the mist of their wet breath, the miasma of
their sweat and the toxic cloud they carried round after a sneeze
or cough, carried the threat of hospital, of experimental and
uncertain treatment. The Joggers did not appear to act after
considering the consequences of proximity. Perhaps they
believed that, having demonstrated their health in so conspic-
uous and panting a way, they could have nothing to do with
public-health matters. Those matters were being talked about
only to inconvenience them. We spoke to some of the Joggers
sharply, as they brushed past us, running up from behind.
They would never acknowledge that they had been spoken to.
We were in a different sphere of experience, speakers of a
different language, movers at so removed a pace that to them
we could not be communicated with. I hated them with an
energy that afterwards was hard to account for.

When the heavy slapping tread of another passed out of our
region of safety, the coffin-length circumference within which
we might have been safe, the word *intubation* would come to
me. The word had been unfamiliar, and now it was everywhere.
It was the invention of some doctor/administrator somewhere;
to put a tube in; to intubate, a scientist's foolish idea of how
words should work, as if the verb *to eat* would be better
expressed as *infoodate*. The word *intubate* was an uncaring and
sinister neologism, the imbecile invention of someone who
knew no better and cared nothing for language. The word had
no life of its own, as words should have, with contradictory
and secret meanings hidden within it, as *contradict* fights
against a word and *seminaries* plant a seed. When a Jogger
pushed past us, spraying sweat and spittle, the word came to
me. Such people cared nothing for language, or only that one
should call them *runners* and not *joggers*, their interest solely
solipsistic. When we reached home, shaken with the stress of

And now I had to think. She was wonderfully composed, that girl, and the drinks she would bring in should contribute to that composure. She would want them to. I thought of Hofmannsthal's Arabella, his libretto for Richard Strauss ending with his heroine descending the staircase holding a single glass of water. Sadie had never heard of Hofmannsthal, but she would want to enter with the same slight but daunting dignity as that. She could not enter the front room with beer for everyone; she could not enter, however, with a single can or bottle or glass; she would not stoop to distinguishing one of these old people. I puzzled; I went over the possibilities. For a mad moment I wondered whether it would seem patronizing to state as a fact that Sadie would never have heard of Hofmannsthal. Perhaps I should make her a devotee of German Jugendstil poetry. But no. She had never heard of Hofmannsthal. And now what Sadie might do herself. I saw –

She was holding a tray, looking down modestly at the laminated picture on it, of a cottage in a rose-thick garden, and on the tray were three unopened cans of beer. Sadie had delighted the family since she was tiny by bringing a beer to her father or uncle, by lighting his cigarette, by learning the word *fuck*; she was a handmaiden to adulthood, and knew just how it was done. There was satire as well as dignity in her use of a tray for the beers.

My dad sent me, she said. Have a Carlsberg. They're delicious.

Neil took one. But now he was standing and did not know how to sit down again.

Good girl, one of the men said.

Glad you're here, aren't you, Neil said. Your mum's birthday.

Glad I'm here, Sadie said. She threw her head back; she laughed. In her T-shirt and black tracksuit bottoms, she was learning about her power. Neil would do.

She's got a boyfriend, I hear, Neil said.

Please, please, it isn't such a story, she has only a … Gio's mother said.

They grow up so fast, one of the men said comfortably. I remember the day this one was born, and her mother, too.

Sadie took the man's plate from his lap, reaching down without hesitation. He made no move. She took a bite from his pork pie; small, ladylike, quick. She went to return the plate to his crotch, but he was too fast for her, lifting his hands to take it.

I remember the day you had your wife put down, Sadie said, stepping back. Pulled the plug on her, didn't you.

There's no need for that, the man said, not raising his voice. Bringing my Mary into it.

It's their age, Neil said.

It's my age, Sadie said, leaning back against the wall. He likes my age, this one. Likes looking at me, don't you.

I thought you liked older men, Neil said. His voice was forced and jocular. The others looked at him. Boyfriend of twenty-five, I heard.

Drink your beer, you dickhead, Sadie said. And take a good look, because I'm going now. Did you hear that?

She put her head out of the door and shouted towards the kitchen. I'm going, she shouted. That's Andy now. I'm sick of this. Wheeled out for your friends. I've got my whole life. I've had it. I've fucking had it.

That was what I had seen, those last words, and the summoned boyfriend in the blue car. I heard nothing more, not even the exit of the guests from the illegal party. They must have gone by the time the police came round. They came round not on account of Gio breaking the rules but because he had called them. And in a few hours a small story had appeared in the local newspaper online: a girl only fifteen had gone missing, and a photograph of Sadie. *Missing* hardly seemed the word; everyone knew where she was, and who with. The imagination went out to what it could not see, and the scenes constructed until the imagination could no longer bear to do so. Just that small dark figure, almost pushing the girl into his blue car, in impatience and fear, and the girl, wanting it all. And the police came.

Our walks continued, every day, at the same time. Sometimes, in the early days, we had taken our walks individually. Although living and being with my husband did not feel like facing the obligations of company, still we had both valued an hour of real solitude. But in those days we took our walk together without needing to discuss it. We talked, heartlessly, about Sadie. She was gone for four days, and every day we talked about her. Our imaginations reached out. My husband was a romantic, and believed in her being holed up in a paradise of passion.

He's redecorated a bedroom just for her, he said. A heart-shaped bed. Pink walls like the inside of a great big heart. And the walls hung with photographs of the pair of them.

I don't know, I said. I was harder-hearted, and kept in mind that Sadie was some months away from being legally able to sleep with anyone. Romance, I thought, was not to the point, and I constructed some hair-raising fates for the pretty girl.

A dungeon underneath the house, I said. She's been promised a bedroom of her own, but it's actually the cellar, converted. And every so often the doorbell rings, and it's one of his friends …

Oh, come on, my husband said. That's awful. The most he could be persuaded into was a gang of white slavers, kidnapping girls by first seducing them, then shipping them off to Buenos Aires.

But I don't think Argentina is the right destination any more, I said sadly. Perhaps the Gulf, do you think?

Sadie must be regretting the day she ever said hello to that man, my husband said. You must be so happy today.

What do you mean, I said. Oh, because it's raining. Yes, I love a walk in the rain.

I'm glad someone loves it, my husband said.

Sadie's longing to feel the rain on her face, I said. Locked up as she is, as we speak, in a crate labelled St Bernard in the hold of Yemeni Airways, I said. Drugged and silent. She'll be regretting the very day.

But was he acting alone, my husband said, or is there someone behind him, the brains of the organization?

It all happens on the dark web, these days, I said. Neither of us knew what the dark web was; we had once seen a television documentary about it. Information gets passed from one user to another, and nobody will ever be able to track it down. There's a mastermind. It wasn't the boyfriend. It must be the Stalinist. It must be Neil.

Who would ever suspect him, my husband said lightly. We laughed a good deal, walking away from home towards a green space. We were only an hour about our walk. We kept it strictly within the rules. It had been months since we'd even crossed the river, or gone more than a mile from home.

I wish I could write, I said, but fondly.

It will come back, he said, stating a fact.

I think of things, I said. But the texture has gone.

What do you mean, he said.

I did not quite know how to say what I meant. I could only feel, wordlessly, what I meant, and perhaps that was the problem. I had started to write, and everything had held initial possibilities; sometimes the subjects were close at hand, and I had thought about what would happen if the shortages and sickness and silences grew worse, what a day in that world would be like. But there was nothing to look at and no one to listen to, and everything I imagined dried and withered, like plants kept from rain. It will come back, my husband said, and I said the same thing to myself lightly, without much emphasis. And it was true that an idea had come to me, the dream of a journey.

It was raining, but we had put on our waterproofs, a yellow oilskin fisherman's coat and sou'wester for him, a green hooded cape for me, which I had bought, in another life, in Canada. The rain falling through the newly clean air of London, washing the empty roads to a polish and shine, had a joy in it, and we liked to walk through it – me more than my husband, true, but both of us liked it to some degree. The Joggers were gone; as my mother used to say, they must be made of sugar to be put off by a bit of rain. Ten minutes after leaving home, the weight of the summer downpour increased, and we stood under a tree until the worst of it had gone by.

What a weight of warm Atlantic water, I said, quoting a favourite poem by Ted Hughes.

It's a good shelter, a pomelo tree, my husband said. He was right. I had not registered, but we were beneath Marianne's pomelo trees, cut neatly to allow pedestrians to pass by unhindered – I dare say a solution accepted unwillingly by *the man from the Council*. That weight of warm Atlantic water had crashed into Marianne's father's orchard in Grenada, and had swung back to wash her London pomelos and remind them of where they came from. The day was dark and the rain was heavy. Marianne did not come out to greet us, and in any case the fruit of her tree was long since taken away. In some minutes the rains slowed, and we went on; very quickly, almost in a burst of temperament, a silver blaze of light on the wet pavement. The sun had emerged. We lowered our hoods and walked on. Today we would walk around the common, and see if we could find the alder we had read about. We would smell the elderflower after the rain and squelch across the large stretch of lawn. We would take our time, and enjoy the clean wet emptiness that discouraged the Joggers, with their eyes fixed on their little watches, thinking only of themselves, not noticing when they were running through an avenue of London plane trees, and when along a path bounded by cherry trees in full blossom, past a line of lime trees making the air heady with perfume. We would do what the Joggers would never do: stop, and wait, and raise our hoods when it rained; we would take pleasure in looking, and talk some more at length and with amusement about what Sadie's boyfriend could have done with her.

Our street was mostly straight, and when we turned into it we saw immediately that there was a police car in the middle of the wet road outside Gio's house. A kind of impasse had been reached in a situation. In a reflex, we slowed down. Something was happening of great violence, but happening at no speed at all. If we were too fast, or even moved at an ordinary pace, we would have to go inside before the drama got any further. Neil was standing in his open doorway watching – I wanted to say with his mouth open. Outside Gio's house were his sister Rosa, brother-in-law and their son. Sadie was there, too, still sitting in the car, evidently having been returned by the police. Had she insisted on being returned to her uncle's house rather than her own? Or was it just that he had been the one talking to the police? All of them were shouting. One policeman was still at the wheel. The other, a policewoman, was standing by the open back door of the car. We approached regretfully, pretending to take an interest in small things lying on the pavement, affecting to tell each other stories so interesting that we had to stop walking altogether. The situation seemed to be stuck. The girl had been returned by the police, but protesting all the way, and now was refusing to leave the police car. What her brother was shouting at her could not have encouraged her: he was calling her a *stupid little tart* and worse. From time to time he made a small dash forward. Each time he did so, Gio laid a calming index finger on his forearm. Everyone was soaked with the falling rain, like the last scene of a film.

How this situation would ever reach an end was not clear. From time to time, the police officer's radio would crackle into life, and she would speak briefly into it. Her impatience was obvious. This had been going on for less than an hour – there had been no sign of it when we had left the house – but perhaps not much less than that. We approached our house unwillingly. The rain had been heavy, but was now coming to an end. Neil theatrically held a hand out from where he stood, in his doorway, and raised his face to the sky, not interested in the weather, but performing the role of a man who is interested in it. He now crossed the road, still maintaining an air of casualness, and sat down on our front wall, the better to watch the situation unfold.

That's too much, my husband said. We were only a hundred yards from the drama.

He thinks he's got a chance now the boyfriend's thrown her out, I said.

You don't know that, he said. I'm going to ask him if he wants me to go and get him some popcorn.

Now the policewoman raised her hands and dropped them again. She, too, was performing an emotion, exasperation, and washing her hands of the consequences. Perhaps the police felt they had been misled into a missing-person investigation when the girl had just gone off with her boyfriend without permission. At any rate, the substance of the drama was now at an end. Her brother walked forward with purpose. He took his sister's legs where she sat in the back of the police car, and started to drag. Sadie began to scream. The police officer stood

leaning on her service vehicle, unmoved. Stuart came forward.
He had never had a role to perform, as far as we could see, but
now, masterfully, he took on a role. I admired it; I saw for the
first time what had drawn Gio to him. He could see that if the
girl's brother took her out by her feet, she would fall and bang
her head on the pavement. Her brother would not care; in a
paroxysm of rage, he was shouting at her. She was a stupid
little tart; underage whore; paedos' plaything; and it went on.
I enjoyed *paedos' plaything*. I thought it had a real zing to it,
and committed it to memory. Out she came, like a mermaid,
her feet together in her brother's grip, and Stuart taking her
shoulders in his big dependable gardener's hands. Gio was
almost smiling; he could see that everything would be all right,
now Stuart had taken charge. She waved her hands around,
shouting. What she was shouting was *I'm not your, I'm not your*,
the exact terms of the humiliation failing her. Now we were at
our door. I gave Neil, who was sitting on our wall, a disapproving look. I would not speak to him. But it turned out that he
would speak to me. He looked up, his face bright with lust and
possibility.

What a fuck-up, he said.

I ignored him – I gave him a full-scale Victorian cut. I
looked directly at him and made no acknowledgement that he
had spoken. The Cut Direct, I know it was termed. My
husband murmured something more generous. We went inside
and shut the door. In the street outside, Sadie was screaming
still. What her boyfriend was doing, I could not guess. He was
nowhere to be seen. Perhaps he was finished with her. Her
brother was still shouting, in rage and a sort of personal
humiliation. Get her in, he was saying. Just fucking get her in
the house. There were, too, Gio's coaxing tones, whether
employed on the police officers, to persuade them everything
was under control, or to talk Sadie into a state of calm. And it

seemed to work. In a moment Stuart said, Much obliged, to the police officers. We'll take it from here. They shut the door. The police officer got into her car. For a few minutes they sat there, writing up their notes on the incident. Then they drove off. In the newly rainless silence outside, a dove nearby insistently purred. A voice was heard. What a fuck-up, the voice said, rattling it off and, it was apparent, not speaking to anyone. The remark was made to the street. Neil got up and went into his house. For him, the story was over once he understood he would never be the hero of it.

I was thinking, my husband said, we haven't had any rice for a while.

A week at least, I said.

Eight days, he said. Would you mind making a curry tonight?

Not at all, I said. A vegetable biriani.

If we can eat early, he said. I'm starving. I've got a meeting at four. But then I'm free.

That would be perfect, I said. I'll make some raita, too.

But neither of us moved. We were not looking at each other, but as we were looking in the same direction, out of the window, our gazes somehow held each other peaceably. The silence in the street pulsed, coagulated into a sound; the sound padded, slapped heavily. It was the Jogger. He was returning. He passed out of our view in a second, perspiring, purple, his eyes full of accumulated blood. The sound had risen, taken a specific form, and now started to diminish. I knew what was happening. He ran, slowing, and he reached the house twenty houses from ours. The front door was painted a dark navy blue. He fumbled in his pocket, panting, for his house keys. But they were not there.

Oh, God, he murmured.

The end of a, he said.

Why does this, he said.

He leant his forehead against the paintwork. It was cool against his hot wet face. He could feel the layer of skin intervening between bone and wood, that was all. He felt like giving up.

They are inside the house, he said, trying to calm himself.

The door opened. He stood upright and did not fall.

The boy was in the doorway. His face formed a question.

Thank you, William, the man said. He placed a damp hand on the boy's head. Together they went inside. The door was shut.

TWO

FREE INDIRECT STYLE

1

The father was walking down the stairs in his house. There were five flights between the top floor and the cellar. Four of the flights were carpeted, an even dark blue colour, and two of the flights now had a slowly rising chair attached. He had reached the middle of the flight between ground floor and landing. A movement under his moccasins made him pause. The carpet had shifted under his tread a tenth of an inch. He gripped the banister firmly and went a few steps further down, turning to inspect what had happened. The carpet was held in place by brass stair rods, and one had become loose. The father lowered himself onto his knees. It was a job he would have done in ten minutes five years ago. It ought to be seen to straight away. That sort of thing could be very dangerous. It would be as well to get somebody to take a look at all the stair rods at the same time. When one went, others would follow. They had done a good job, those stair rods; they had been in place quietly for forty years.

2

The mother sat in the chair. It was comfortable, but her back ached a little. She wriggled. She must have been here in the chair for some time. It was a room that she knew. There were two vases of flowers in front of the fireplace. The fire was not lit, but the room was quite warm. There were pictures on the walls. There was a painting of some garlic, spring onions and a red onion, and over the fireplace, a painting of a river in a landscape. The word *Derbyshire* came to her. Her mouth was dry, but there was a glass of water by her, on a side table. She took that. There was a photograph on it, too, of a man smiling and looking up as he signed a book. Next to him was another man with his hand on his shoulder. It was a lovely photograph, and the mother remembered that it was her son on his wedding day. She put the glass of water down. There was a nice smell, a smell of polish and flowers, but there was no smell of onions or garlic. One day there used to be smells of onion and garlic and there was a picture of them.

The room was in shades of purple; the walls were mauve, the carpet a deeper purple. The curtains, which ran round the bay window, were a dark tweedy purple, as tall as the room. What big curtains! Someone had had a job putting those up and sewing them. She would not have liked to have had that job. It was lovely to look through the windows edged with purple and see the different greens of the garden, and the flowers too. It must be summer, the weather was so nice. But then she looked again, and it was not green at all. It was only one tree that was green, and the others were all bare branches. It was a blue-sky day but it must be cold outside. That was what sometimes happened.

The ceiling of the room was beautiful. It was a pattern in plaster, weaving in and out like ribbons. This was her house, and her husband's too. When they had looked for a house to buy, it had been this ceiling that had made her say, This one. And she liked it just as much now. She thought it might be time to go to bed. Her back was aching and she had been in this chair for a long time. She called out.

In a moment the father came in. He was holding a phone, and looking bothered.

It's a lovely room, this one, she said.

Can I get you something, he said. I was just trying to call Sam, but he's not answering.

What are we having for lunch, she said.

You've just had lunch, he said, quite crossly. I cooked you some fish and vegetables. It was only an hour ago. Don't you remember?

Oh, yes, she said. She was not hungry but she did not remember. This is a lovely room, she said. When we first came here to look, it was the ceiling that sold the house to me. I came in here and I said, What a beautiful ceiling. I've always liked it.

Do you want your book, the father said.

Yes, please, she said. There was a book on the table in front of her. I've always liked reading, she said. It's the thing I like to do more than anything. I've always been a great reader.

I know, the father said. Here's your book. I'm just in the other room.

He went out, closing the door. She looked at the cover of the book she was holding. She knew this book. It was a book by her son. She started to read it. Her son had written a lot of books and this was one of them. In a while she turned the page. A figure walked past the window outside, through the front garden. There was a clatter in the front hallway, of the letterbox opening and shutting again, and a heavy thud as something fell onto the carpet. A figure walked past the window outside. She thought it might be the postman. On her lap was an open book. She was on the second page, but she was not quite sure how much she had read. She turned back a page and started to read from the beginning.

You can always read a good book more than once, she said to herself, and her big sister was telling her in her bossy way that she would never meet a nice boy, sitting in the corner reading a book all the time. That had been a long time ago. She wondered what her sister was doing now. The man in the photograph on the table next to her was her son, who had written a lot of books. On her lap was a book that was open. She turned it back to the cover, and saw that the book she was reading was a book by her son. She knew she had read it before but it didn't matter. You can always read a good book more than once, she said to herself.

3

The wife of the builder had failed to make a success of her morning. She had got out of bed and seen that her first meeting was in only ten minutes, at eight o'clock. She left her husband still in bed. He didn't have to do anything today, or any other day. He could get his children some breakfast, or they could get it themselves.

She went to the bathroom; she brushed her hair quickly and impatiently; she washed her face and put on a dark green blouse and yesterday's skirt, which no one would see. Then she took a cup of instant coffee into the study, shut the door and logged on to her first meeting.

There was a list of things that should have been achieved by the team. She'd made a list of these things the night before. She was the third to appear; Sanjay and Anna were already there, and then two more quickly turned up. They had to wait five minutes for the last of them. The builder's wife engaged them in conversation about how they were finding working from home, and how they had been filling their days. It was important, she told them, to take time out and to enjoy their leisure. The conversation was a bit slow and stilted. The builder's wife thought they might be a little unsure about what the rules were now. The first two at the meeting had been talking in an easy, relaxed way when she had logged on. Then it had dried up. She made a little joke about the difficulties of working productively with children in the house. She explained, as she had explained before, that she was talking about her husband's children from his first marriage. They were grown up and the toddler training was only needed for her husband, these days. They laughed a bit at that. One of them made a sort of face. She didn't know why.

In five minutes the kid showed up and gave a cursory apology. He was the same age as the builder's daughter, and straight out of university. Pretty easy to find that you could do your first graduate-trainee post from your parents' spare bedroom and not have to worry about travelling or work clothes. The last time they'd met, she'd been a bit tough on him. Today he had done one of those editing jobs on his backdrop that the kids liked so much. He wasn't sitting in a small room in front of bookcases, like the others, and as he had done last time. He appeared to be in a magnificent modernist apartment. It looked like a photograph from a lifestyle magazine. She made a comment on it. It was just an image, he explained. Another of the team said sarcastically that they could see that. Then the trainee said that it was for some degree of privacy. After all, he said, you wouldn't expect your supervisors in normal circumstances to be able to look at and pass judgement on your home.

The others in the team were quiet. A bad-taste remark that might have professional consequences. The builder's wife remarked lightly that of course they all felt like that, but it just had to be lived with. She remembered that the last time they had met, the same quiet at a bad-taste remark had fallen when she had said something about the trainee's backdrop. It had not been the backdrop of a boy of twenty-two, but one you had when you were middle-aged, with a line of hardback books and some of those objects that fell under the category of *ornament*, she forgot what. He was in his mum's spare room and now, apparently, he was in some expensive Swiss chalet. Screw them. She didn't like them anyway and in six months this contract would be done and she would never see them again. Now they had all shown up, she started running through the list of things to do, typing them up in the comments sidebar for those responsible to copy and paste. She was in her study, with dark green wallpaper and solid furniture. Behind her was a stained-oak bookshelf of clearly labelled grey box files, covering the years from 2008–9 to 2020–21. That was what this team would see in the background of the team leader on Zoom. They would not see its history, that the shelves had been built and the walls papered by a builder she had called in fifteen years ago, who had explained that he was recently divorced with two small children. She was satisfied with the limits of what they would see.

Outside the room a voice rose. *Mop*, it said. One of the others was talking, the IT planner, explaining the costs and benefits of the two proposed routes. This woman knew her stuff and needn't be interrupted to seek clarification. The builder's wife tapped the *mute* button. She called out briskly. Not now, she said. *Mop* was the word that the children had settled on for her, naturally continuing to call their mother *Mum*, and she answered to it.

He's eaten the last yogurt, the voice said.

I was hungry, another voice said.

You promised I could have that yogurt, the builder's daughter said. That was mine.

The delivery's coming tomorrow, the builder's wife shouted, not taking her attention from the computer screen.

But I want it now, the builder's daughter said, her voice rising.

But I want it now, the builder's son said, mimicking her. Mmm, that yogurt, that lovely hazelnut yogurt, it was so delicious, I loved it so much.

Mop, the builder's daughter said, almost wailing.

The builder's wife switched the computer's audio back on. She said, briskly, One second, please, before turning off both audio and vision. She got up and opened the door. Outside in the hallway were the builder's children. Both were unwashed, giving off a smell of sleep, their hair tousled. The builder's son was leaning on the piano that had been in the hallway for years, having been taken ultimately from the builder's childhood home. Nobody had found a better place for it. There was a banana skin growing black on the open dusty keyboard. It, too, had been there some time, though perhaps not years. On the floor of the hallway lay a tangle of four people's shoes, his, hers, hers, his.

I'm in a very important meeting, she said.

It's always the same, Mop, the builder's daughter said. It's not fair.

How old are you? the builder's son said. You sound like you're seven.

Go and bother your father, the builder's wife said. I'm far too busy. If you can't wait until tomorrow when the food's coming, try and persuade him to drive you into town to go to Waitrose.

We had to queue in the rain for forty minutes last time we went to Waitrose, the builder's daughter said. It's not fair. I hate this. I hate it.

Well, that's life, the builder's wife said. I don't want to hear another word.

She went back inside the study, shutting the door with firmness. On the screen the five members of the team were no longer talking, waiting for her to return. She could see that one of them – the IT woman – had her lips pursed. It was too bad. These things happened and people should just be more understanding.

I'm sorry about that, the builder's wife said, switching her camera and microphone on once more. If you could just run through the salient points once more, Amber –

That was what it said on the bottom of the little box on the screen, *Amber*. There was no difficulty these days in remembering the names of members of the team.

– I'd be eternally grateful. Important that we're all on the same page.

Singing from the same hymn sheet, the graduate trainee said, from his fake Swiss chalet. She wondered whether she would, after all, be able to speak positively about this one's contribution when the time came.

4

The builder woke when the builder's wife got up. She banged around the bedroom like a herd of wildebeest. Making a point. As per usual. Then she drew the curtains and went off to the meeting she'd been going on about at dinner last night. The builder got up. This house never seemed totally his. Being moved in. He was buggered if he'd get up just for the sake of it because he'd had the morning let in on him and because some people thought you ought to be doing stuff to keep yourself busy.

You weren't allowed to do anything anyway. The government wasn't allowing it. He was on furlough and all the team were on furlough and not his to worry about. He got up, but only to close the curtains and go back to bed. He had a bit more of the old shut-eye. *The team*: what she'd persuaded him to start calling them. He couldn't remember what he used to call them before he walked through the door of number 37 Peshawar Road, to give a lady a quote for a study that wanted decorating. It would be *staff* next. Soon he slept. He dreamt about scoring a goal in a match. In his dream, he ran like he was seventeen, running like he was swept away in an irresistible flood.

It was after ten when he woke up again. Better get up before he found himself in the doghouse. Nothing to do. The books were all square and checked, the furlough payments all running nicely, the regulations saying you couldn't go anywhere or do anything, not likely to be going anywhere soon. He reckoned he'd just potter about today.

He thought he'd better check the email, though, and sat up in his pyjamas to look. Buried in an avalanche of bumf was an email from Waitrose. The order had been amended. Not by him it hadn't. He didn't know why – it was probably just something had been left off – but he checked. Glad he did.

What's all this then, he said, in the sitting room. The builder's daughter and the builder's son were lolling on the sofa and armchair, the boy's legs over the far arm of the yellow armchair, the girl at full length. The TV was on. It was one of those programmes about buying houses in Portugal.

Yeah, the builder's daughter said. Her attention was fixed.

Who put this in the Waitrose order, he said.

What, the girl said.

I told you, the boy said. You're in for it now.

Look at this, the builder said. He read out the first five lines of the order, which were nothing special. Then he got to the bit where somebody had ordered sixty honey and ginger yogurts, sixty hazelnut, and sixty caramel.

I like caramel yogurt, the girl said. It's really nice.

That's nearly two hundred yogurts, the builder said.

She doesn't want to run out, the boy said.

You're an idiot, the builder said. I've cancelled them all and I'm getting her to change the password on my computer.

What, you cancelled them all? the girl said. But we've got to have some yogurts. He finished the last one this morning and that one was meant for me. Why have you cancelled them. It's not fair.

We don't want two hundred yogurts, the builder said. One, you can't eat them all, and, two, I'm not made of money.

I think what she means is – the builder's son said. Look, they're going for the bungalow on the Algarve. Ew. I think what she means is that there were ten yogurts on the order anyway and she just added a few more but now there aren't any.

Well, I'll put them back, then, the builder said.

It's too late now, the builder's son said. You have to make any changes before ten thirty the day before. You just came in time, cancelling the yogurts. No yogurts for you.

Not the end of the world, the builder said. He had just saved himself, what, a hundred and thirty quid and the kids would go hungry.

He went into the kitchen. He made himself a cup of coffee – instant coffee, he couldn't be bothered with the espresso machine this morning. All the time a voice was rising in the other room. If this sort of thing went on much longer, he reckoned he'd spend the day going round the rolling acres. Half an acre the house had. It didn't sound like much but it was a hell of a job to take care of, the borders she'd had put in, the wall of black bamboo at the end that was always making a bid for freedom, the water feature that had broken down and wouldn't be fixed until things changed. Half an acre, though. That was two thousand square metres, which was forty metres by forty metres or more realistically twenty metres by eighty metres or maybe ten metres by twenty or – his mind went on into the realms of remote fantasy – a corridor of a garden fifty centimetres wide and a kilometre long. Say in reality twenty by eighty, something like that. It was an ordinary suburban garden, but they were close to the edge of the city, and the wildlife were moving in. Once, the kids had seen a sheep that had got in somehow. The first year after they got married, they'd planted three hundred tulip bulbs. Spent a week choosing them from a catalogue, took three days from Friday to Sunday planting them, and on Monday morning woke to see something had dug them all up and eaten them. Badgers, apparently.

The voice was still going on in the other room. He looked out of the window. The sun was shining, out there in the garden. Would be good if you could just switch stuff off. That would be an improvement. He didn't have one solitary thing to do today. It wasn't just the yogurt, the voice was insisting, not just about yogurt.

5

The builder's daughter lay on the sofa. She clutched the remote control in the certainty of power.

It's not about the yogurt, she said.

It is about the yogurt, her brother, the builder's son said. If there was yogurt you wouldn't be going on about it.

You ate the last one, she said.

It was yummy, he said. It was caramel.

It was not caramel, the builder's daughter said. The caramel ones always get eaten first and then the hazelnut and then the honey and ginger. It was definitely honey and ginger.

Just think of that yummy caramel yogurt I had, the builder's son said. But now there's no more yogurt for at least a week.

Ken seems to be sold on the three-bedroom villa, the warm voice on the television said. But Jennifer has some concerns about the access road.

Well, that's fine, the builder's daughter said. I can manage perfectly well without.

She sat up and put her feet down. On the table in front of her there were two mugs, three plates, a bowl with a half-centimetre of brown milk, the remains of a breakfast that had started two hours ago. There were also a small glass swan, a wooden duck, a dark blue vase and a china cat smoking a pipe. The builder's daughter placed the plates together, then the bowl on top, and the mugs to one side with their handles facing the same direction. Then she moved the four objects so that they were in a line across the table, arranged in order of size, the swan, the cat, the duck, the vase. The table was dusty but that was better.

I can't see now, the builder's son said. You've put that sock-ing great vase in the way.

Sorry! the builder's daughter sang, and moved the vase to the right, to the edge of the table. She moved the duck and the cat too, so that they would be the same distance from each other.

Still can't see, the builder's son said, but contentedly.

Do you remember when we got this, the builder's daughter said.

What, the builder's son said.

This! the builder's daughter said, putting her finger on the china cat. He was such an idiot not knowing what she was talking about. Don't you remember? We got it with her.

Oh, yeah, the builder's son said.

You were such a baby, the builder's daughter said. It was years ago. She said, What are you getting Daddy for Christmas and we didn't have any ideas.

Where was that place, the builder's son said.

It was that place where we used to go when Granny came, the builder's daughter said. You know.

No idea, the builder's son said. I remember buying it, though.

You remember that, the builder's daughter said. You chose the cat and I said I liked it too. Then she says, Well, if you think that's what Daddy would like, here's the money.

She hands over the dosh, the builder's son said.

She gave you eighty pounds, the builder's daughter said. It's seventy-five pounds, that stupid cat. I don't know why we thought that was the sort of thing Daddy was longing for, for his Christmas present. And you just look at the money in your hand and you say –

I can't remember what I said, the builder's son said.

You want to know if she would just give you the money and then you can buy him something cheaper and keep the rest of the money. Like buy him a pencil sharpener or something.

A pencil sharpener, the builder's son said. Now that would have been a good present. He'd have used that, probably, not some stupid china cat.

But you're basically saying to her, Can you give me seventy-five pounds. To your new mother.

To Mop, the builder's son said, with contempt, making quotation marks in the air in front of him. That makes a lot of sense, the builder's son said. Asking her for the money. And he didn't want it anyway and now I think it's kind of hideous.

I really like it, the builder's daughter said.

She ought to be applying for jobs today, she supposed. The list of trainee schemes that she'd made with Mop was printed out and waiting for her to sit down and do something about it. That had been two weeks ago, though. All those different futures! They had been organized in order of closing date – Mop had done that – and she had an awful feeling that some of the ones at the beginning were now closed. She didn't really think it mattered. Everyone got a job one way or another and, anyway, she hadn't sat down with Mop who would help her to write a good application letter and some of them wanted to know why you wanted to work for blah-di-blah, which she often couldn't think of an answer to. If the worst came to the worst she could do Daddy's paperwork, the stuff that Mop did now and complained that she wasn't there to work for him for nothing, she had her own stuff to get on with.

There was no reason why they couldn't go to Waitrose in any case and get some yogurts. She would go herself if Mop would lend her the car or she could just get Mop to drive her there after last time. It just wasn't fair that he had eaten the last one when he'd known that one was meant for her, and because he'd been stupid and they'd laughed about it, mucking about on Daddy's computer, it had ended up with all the yogurts that were supposed to be coming tomorrow not coming at all.

It looked as if the sun was shining outside. She couldn't tell if it was the sort of sun that was cold or the other sort. The last time she had gone outside was about a week ago. There was nothing to go outside for. Literally all her friends were like a hundred miles away. Caroline had WhatsApped the group yesterday saying that her parents made her go out for a walk for an hour every day and everyone had sent that vomiting emoji. Not even into the garden. She was going to tell Mop that the whole locked-up thing was sending her like totally insane and the only thing that could possibly cure her from the insanity and bipolar depression and probably cutting herself in the end would be to get in the car and drive to Waitrose to buy some yogurts. And when Mop objected that they'd had to wait in a queue outside Waitrose last time for an hour, she'd say that if she loved her then she'd do this little thing. No, a better idea: that if she did it then they'd sit down this evening and write all those applications for trainee schemes together.

I hate this crap, her brother said.

Some doubts are creeping into Jennifer's mind, the voice on the screen said. And they go beyond questions about rights of access.

I don't know why we agreed to move to Portugal, the woman in the programme said. I think it was Ken's idea and I just went along with it.

It's crap, the builder's daughter said.

6

The Prince of Wales was in Wandsworth. The visit had not been announced, apart from to those whom it most concerned. They had been civilly asked not to spread the word beyond their closest family. A crowd should in no circumstances be allowed to gather. In these circumstances, the man on the telephone had gone on to say. Abdullah had thought that you should probably not say that something should happen *in no circumstances* and then qualify it by saying *in these circumstances*. He said nothing, however. And now the Prince of Wales was approaching his little delicatessen, Alfredo's. They had managed to stay open until now. Abdullah practised his sentences, although he knew his English after twenty years was as good as anyone could ask for. His wife stood behind the counter, a new and girlish ribbon in her hair. The little boy, Harry, had been coaxed into a bow tie and stood by his father's side in the doorway, underneath hanging hams, baskets of gleaming aubergines, peppers, three sorts of tomatoes, and a positive thicket of pineapples. It was wonderful that this man was visiting his little shop. He would be King one day. Both Abdullah and Harry were being as good as gold, standing patiently.

And then the Prince of Wales was there, very red-faced, as if he had too much blood for one person, but smiling and joyous.

How marvellous, he said. What an extraordinarily tempting shop you have. Are you Alfredo?

I am Alfredo, Your Royal Highness, said Abdullah. But only in a manner of speaking. My name is Abdullah, and this is my son, Harry. I have always loved the food of Italy.

It truly is a marvellous thing, the Prince said. Hello, there, young man. And what wonderful things you have here, I can see. Tell me – how have things been over the last months?

It is true that we have had many several difficulties, Abdullah said. He could have *bit his tongue*. He was correcting himself; he said *many* without thinking, and then went for *several* as more optimistic. But he had said something that sounded like an Iraqi bumpkin off the plane.

Ah, yes, the Prince said, his face quickly sombre.

Which we are contriving to overcome, Abdullah said. The Prince started to thank him. Abdullah put his hand out; the Prince without hesitation did the same, and they shook. Then he was away.

I have plenty of photographs, Wendy said. We can have one framed behind the counter. You weren't supposed to touch him. They were very clear about that.

The crowd had moved on; they seemed to be alone, the three of them.

Always, always the Prince will remember the idiot who was told not to touch him and who shook his hand, Abdullah said. And the fellow who said he had *many several difficulties*.

He put his hands to his face in despair.

Well, that won't show up in the photo, Wendy said. What you said to him. I wouldn't give it another thought.

7

The builder's wife had given in, in the end. You had to do everything yourself. The builder was down the bottom of the garden. His kids were bored and kicking up a row that showed no sign of letting up. The easiest thing was to give in and take her to Waitrose to buy the idiotic yogurts. She cut the meeting short – people did have family emergencies, after all – and told them the afternoon might start off a bit late. The lunchtime queue at Waitrose was long; it was also strange, not much like a line. Everyone was six feet behind the one in front and six feet ahead of the one behind. The woman in front had hissed at the builder's daughter when she blundered a few feet closer; they had discussed her after that animatedly. But finally the yogurts were bought. They came home. The builder's daughter settled on the sofa for an afternoon that would be rather like the morning, pushing the builder's son over. The builder was said to be in the shed. She started her meeting an hour late.

The email arrived an hour after that, from the company's director of tech.

Need a quick word at 6 today
I was hoping to log off by then
Won't take long

And then an invitation arrived without any more being said. She went back to her meeting.

How's it going, the man said. He was brisk, early thirties, in a big tasteful space that she had no reason to believe was simulated. Childless, she would have said. She had asked him once directly; he had looked back at her levelly for a good five seconds before saying that he preferred to keep things on a professional level with contractors as well as colleagues. She had never met him in person. The first meetings, setting the whole thing up, had been with his predecessor. She had moved on. He had a shaved head, glinting glasses, and what might have been an Australian accent. His name was Scott. Behind him on a blank white wall a large blue painting, a bookcase full of books.

Fine, she said briskly. No need to drag things out after six.

I'll come to the point, he said, and did so. He had dates and times of the incidents raised. That was what he called them. He had checked against the records of online meetings and found them to be correct. The schedule as agreed last year was not being kept to. No: it was true that some disruption would be expected in present circumstances but he did not agree that this delay was unavoidable. He had a definition of *family emergency*, which had never come to her attention. It was, he agreed, a definition that the company had decided on rather than a legally enforceable one. But a template, widely agreed, he believed. He read the definition again.

I think the members of your staff who are complaining – she said, keeping her voice low and reasonable.

Not complaining, he said. Raising issues of justifiable concern. Calling people *complainers* relegates legitimate concerns to the status of stigma.

Does it now, she said, not really caring how that sounded. People recited pretentious rubbish at you they'd read on a flip-chart or PowerPoint at some HR awayday.

I'm not going to discuss how we've become aware of these issues.

I think they don't understand what it is to have children at home, she said. Emergencies arise.

I remember, at one point, he said, you did offer without being asked that they were not your children, that your husband took charge of his own children, and that they were now adults, in any case.

Emergencies arise, she said. I don't think I would have said that I didn't take any responsibility for my husband's children.

We are certainly very sympathetic to different situations, he said. But over the last six weeks meetings have been cancelled or delayed between two and four times every week. I think if this goes on we would like to start discussing possible solutions.

One fucking yogurt, and she was going to lose the project or have to suck up the costs of that anorexic idiot Barbara coming in to supervise everything, with her keen-as-mustard look and her nervous laugh of agreement.

Let's see how it goes, she said, without going into unnecessary details

Yes, I'm not enquiring into your domestic circumstances, he said, as I wouldn't expect to be asked about mine.

That was a nasty one.

I think I can promise that the circumstances – she emphasized the word, putting into it as much of the children as she could, as much of the education at boarding schools, costing hundreds of thousands, and the products now lying on the sofa doing nothing, a husband, a garden that wanted ceaseless attention and labour, all that obligation and blunt human need for yogurt or laundry or the issuing or acceptance of instructions, all that going into the word *circumstances* – have now been resolved and are, I can safely say, in short, now past their most challenging point.

We're not going to see as much of this crap, he said. In short.

I don't know that I would use, she said. She could feel her voice rising.

We'll take a look again in a week, he said. Don't discuss this with the team. I'll talk to them if needed.

It would be needed. There was the ghost of a movement behind him, but whether man or woman, lover or husband, cleaner or colleague, shadow or flesh, she couldn't say. He pursed his mouth, his forehead furrowed. It was a bit like the face someone made when they didn't know what button to press on the computer. But he knew what button to press on the computer. *Has left the meeting*, the screen said. She pressed the button too. There was no one to be informed that she had left and she had the unpleasant feeling that she had not had the last word there. She needed a drink and then dinner, cooked by someone who wasn't her.

8

The son had left the house on his morning walk. The son's husband went with him. *The Morning Walk* by Gainsborough. It was an idyllic morning. The sky was absolutely blue, and quite empty of the sky's usual traffic. They had turned left out of their front door rather than right; the common today rather than the park.

What the hell time did you get up, the husband said.

Must have been half six, the son said.

You're crazy, the husband said, but comfortably. It was now half past nine. The son had woken up with an idea that could not wait, or so he had thought – a dream had gone by with a fully worked-out plot, a matter of desires being raised and frustrated, a secret being discovered and reacted to, a villainous dwarf who knew exactly what he was to do and a sidekick who might have been a woman in a fur coat or a tall dog …

All this, he started explaining to the husband as they walked past the Ethiopian church, the vicarage where the Abuna now lived with his wife and sisters, the unattended garden of the vicarage neck high in thistles, all this was quite unusual. The dreams in this time of seclusion had been dull and quotidian, as if the smallest undertaking could satisfy the soul's desire for discovery, triumphs and adventure. Only two days ago he had reported a dream in which a light bulb had failed in a lamp in the drawing room, and he had gone to the cupboard and found the forty-watt bulb that was needed, and replaced it. And here was a dream that appeared like a gift.

Today, I thought, I am going to go straight away to write it down, the son said.

And you had to start at six thirty, the husband said.

Well, exactly, the son said.

They waited on the Queenstown Road, ready to cross, while a single cyclist in Lycra and a helmet approached from three hundred yards away. Hunched over the curving horns of his handlebars, like a matador, faceless, he approached and passed them. Perhaps there had been no reason to wait for him before crossing the road. They were by way of having forgotten how you crossed roads by now.

The only thing, the son's husband said.

I know what you're going to say, the son said.

A dwarf who's a villain and his villainous sidekick, the son's husband said.

Yes, exactly, the son said.

Quite a shift, the son's husband said. From your usual stuff.

My usual stuff, the son said, with amusement.

The son had gone in a still half-sleeping fugue state of mind to the bookcase where he knew an empty notebook was placed, A4, bound in plain black, and afterwards to the blue ceramic pot on the hall table where three green Pentel pens waited. In his pyjamas, he walked in a steady way without shifts of direction or sharp changes of purpose. The dream and the fugue of entrancement held him. There was a desk in the house but he had always written, since he was quite small, on the end of the dining-room table where things could be written quickly and cleared away, where nothing piled up and no pretension or status attached. Long ago he had read of a novelist whose aim was to find himself opening the double doors to his study at the end of a good morning of work, to greet the awed acolytes and disciples and the *team* who had assembled for luncheon. He read it; not what he wanted. He wrote in a black A4 notebook with a green Pentel pen on the end of a dining table and was done by ten. This morning it had returned in a great wave.

But that was an illusion. He had reached the table, and set the notebook down, and sat, still in his pyjamas, and took the smooth, slightly yielding cap of the green pen in his mouth, pulling it off with his teeth. He opened the notebook. Immediately the thought came: a villain? A dwarf? A long-nurtured desire for revenge? A box of emeralds?

It was a box of aquamarines, he had written in mild rebellion against the dream, having always loved aquamarines best of all precious stones. He had debouched them from the beautiful Brazilian tiara the Queen had and hardly ever wore. That was the source of his box of stones. He let his mind flood with the sense of them; the colour of the fresh pure wash of a Bavarian lake edged with gentians, the queer lucidity so distinct from glass, the feel of the edge of one of them, a slight notch and roughness as if torn away by the cutter, the weight, somehow bottom heavy, of half a dozen fat stones in the hand and the quick warmth of them once held; raise them to the face and smell. But there was no smell, and then an implausible odour of sea salt, and then again nothing. *It was a box of aquamarines*, he had written. Beyond that he did not know where to go. There was only some villainous superdwarf in clumping boots and a leather coat that his dream life had thought a good idea.

What did you do, the son's husband said.

Mucked about, the son said.

No, I meant did you write anything, he said.

I thought I was going to, the son said. But in the end I didn't.

So you woke me up at half past six and from then until nine thirty when I woke up and found you on the sofa.

Reading Ivy Compton-Burnett, the son said. I was reading Ivy Compton-Burnett. She's terribly good. I was going to phone my dad but first it was too early and then I got engrossed in the usual mayhem. She would have known what to do with a box of aquamarines.

Is there something going on, the son's husband said. The words *Ivy Compton-Burnett* would, in any case, have put an end to the conversation. But he was talking about the two red engines in the street ahead of them, the yellow-helmeted firemen milling about, the ladder from the one of them fully extended, and a small, bright, beady woman in a long white nightgown standing outside talking to one of the firemen underneath the arc and shelter of her dark-leaved tree, the tree the two of them now knew was a pomelo.

9

The man was in the kitchen of his flat, on the third floor. He peeled three potatoes, and cut them into neat strips. He filled a frying pan with vegetable oil, two inches deep, turned the gas on and pressed the button to light the flame. He left the kitchen and went into the sitting room. After two minutes, the pan of oil burst into flame, a jet six feet high licking the ceiling. After another minute, something cracked loudly. The man returned from the sitting room, where he had been reading a book. He shut the kitchen door quickly, went to his front door and walked as fast as he could down the stairs. On the ground floor, he knocked on his neighbour's door.

What is it, Marianne said.

It's on fire, the third-floor tenant said.

Oh, you stupid, Marianne said, you stupid, stupid man.

She walked up the stairs, dialling 999 on her mobile phone. The door to the man's flat was open. She went in, and then quickly out again, talking on her phone all the while.

You stupid man, Marianne said, to the third-floor tenant. What were you doing? Deep-fat frying at nine o'clock in the morning, what the Heaven's name for?

I wanted some chips, the third-floor tenant said.

You know you're not to do anything but wait for the carers, Marianne said. She bundled him out onto the street. Now you've gone and burnt down the whole building. Put you in prison they should. You wait here, you stupid old man.

She went quickly from door to door in the building. The second-floor tenant was in, and came out, clutching her computer under her arm. The others were at work.

There's Hugo to get as well, the third-floor tenant said.

When the fire engines arrived, he said it again to the man in charge.

He means his neighbour's cat, Marianne said. She stays at home in the flat next door. I don't know why her name is Hugo.

Right, the man in charge said. The ladders began to rise.

There was a small crowd of onlookers and neighbours. A car went by and slowed as it passed; three passengers on the top of a bus going by turned their heads in synchrony to take it in. Marianne started to explain.

That stupid old man, she said. He shouldn't be living on his own. He's a danger. His mind's all shot to pieces. Gets up and thinks, I want some chips. Chips for breakfast. Forgets about the chip pan, whoosh. Now the whole place is on fire. What the Council is doing letting him live there, who knows. The man from the Council, he's better off sorting this stupid old man out, not making idle threats about the beautiful trees people have planted in their own gardens, that is the truth. And the cat! Stuck on the third floor. Burnt to death because of this stupid old man. Fine, fine ginger cat. I tell you, I been here forty years, never a moment's problem, and now this stupid old man, should be in a home, and my house it's going to burn down. Where are his children, I want to know, where are his children?

Dark smoke was piling out of an open window on the third floor. In short order a firefighter was at the window, on top of a ladder. Another four were inside the third-floor tenant's flat. Water was sprayed. In a few minutes the fire was extinguished. The kitchen was blackened, and stinking. Around the stove, objects had taken on new, irregular shapes, dripping with blackened water, like a lagoon at low tide. The hoses continued to play on the ruin. The man in charge went into the house at a signal from above. He walked up the stairs – they were soaked and pouring with water. He took a look round, and returned to street level.

All right to go back in, then, the third-floor tenant said. Only it's Eileen coming today.

Who's going to look after him, the man in charge said.

Oh, no, Marianne said. You're not getting me. Eileen's his carer. She can sort it out.

You can't go back in, the man in charge said to the third-floor tenant. It's not safe. Someone give him a blanket.

What about Hugo, the third-floor tenant said. What's happened to Hugo.

The son and his husband had been standing in the little group of neighbours and onlookers, but now they moved on. The husband was holding an umbrella, although it was not raining. He made a vague circling gesture with the point, just above the pavement, and the people standing outside the building, underneath a pomelo tree overhanging the pavement, moved back. A point had been made and the point had been taken. The son and the husband extricated themselves from what might have been a little crowd, and they walked away.

I forget which way we were going, he said.

That might be as much excitement as we can take for the day, the son said.

I wonder if there are more or less house fires at the moment, the husband said.

It's probably public information, the son said. People are bored and they'll start to think, Why not cook chips rather than buy those oven chips? Slice them and fry them, use up an hour or two.

That man shouldn't be let near a gas hob, the husband said. He almost burnt the place down.

The two men stood to one side and let a pink perspiring Jogger run past.

They never bother to say thank you, the son said. Here we go.

There was an electronic tune from the son's pocket. It was thirteen notes, originally composed by a Spanish guitarist in 1902. The son took his phone out of his pocket and looked at the screen. The tune repeated itself

I'll call later, he said eventually. Let's have our walk first.

10

Arthur's mother Natasha said, There's always some drama with that one.

Sandip, her husband, was washing up after breakfast. They had a dishwasher; Sandip had concluded that washing up was something he enjoyed. He went on with it, contemplatively. The kitchen was at the front of the house. Together, they watched Wendy bustle off, open the car from ten feet away, hop into it and drive off while fastening her seatbelt.

What, Sandip said. Prince Charles coming to their shop?

We'll never hear the last of that, Natasha said. I meant today, could we look after Harry.

What was it, Sandip said.

Oh, I can't even remember, Natasha said. He's a nice little boy, I don't mind.

Not supposed to, Sandip said. Well, anyway.

Arthur was Harry's best friend and Harry was Arthur's best friend. They were in the same class at school and they sat next to each other and did things together at playtime. Harry could remember that. They had got a line of boys together sometimes and marched around, their arms on the next boy along's shoulders and they'd shouted, Who wants to play – WAR. Who wants to play – WAR. It used to be brilliant. That was when there was school. Now there was only coming over to Arthur's house sometimes and that was all there was.

Going on with Crusaders, right, Arthur said, as soon as Harry's mother was gone. They both bounced with impatience, dancing from one foot to the other. Brutus, Arthur's dog, capered around. He loved Crusaders, too.

There were the face-eaters, Harry said. They look like ordinary people.

But they say, Oh, excuse me, you seem to have something on your nose, Arthur said.

They go like this, Harry said. Like they're going to take it off your nose.

But then they, Arthur said. Joyously, their palms fixed on each other's faces, pushing hard. It was a completely new way of fighting and Arthur and Harry had discovered it at the same time. They made small grunting noises. Brutus ran round and round, maddened with joy. The thing was that when you were face-eating the other one with your hand you could feel that there were even bones in someone's face. It was the best thing that anyone had ever thought of and in a minute to show how brilliant it was Arthur's father came in and told them to go out into the garden before they knocked something over.

11

The builder had given way in the face of strong suggestions: he was making what had always been one of his specialities, a sort of meat bake with layers of sliced potatoes – it had gone through different stages over the years. His preparations were detailed and orderly; he had to prepare all the different elements of the dish before any cooking could begin. In successive piles on the work surface were onions, which he had inexpertly diced, carrots and celery in the same condition; cubes of bacon; crushed garlic; slices of potato, a packet of minced beef, two tins of tomatoes, not yet open; a thick oblong of butter and even, in a small bowl, a couple of spoonfuls of flour (the addition of a white sauce, stirred through the meat, was a recent innovation); and finally some milk, which for some reason had been decanted from the bottle in the fridge into a measuring jug. Just now he was pouring boiling water from the kettle into a second measuring jug that contained a stock cube.

The builder's wife watched him. This sense of orderly preparation in all things had once drawn her to him, and now drove her slightly insane. Everything in his life had to be prepared for; oil and tyre pressure checked before any journey of more than fifty miles; sex had to have all the accoutrements in place before any spontaneity could, with planning, emerge. She reflected that his preparation for cooking was irritating her; so, too, would the alternative, that she had to cook the dinner after her day on the screen. He had no notion that she was being irritated. His concentration was total. That was what was allowing him to ignore the third person in the kitchen, his daughter. She had been talking for some time now.

She had seen a film on the television that afternoon, an old film, and had been explaining the plot since the slicing of the onions, ten minutes ago. The reproduction of a narrative was not one of her strengths.

And then the mother came out, and she hadn't seen her daughter in thirty years, so of course they don't recognize each other at first. This is in the South of France – the daughter's gone to live there. She's got a daughter now too, she's almost grown-up, in the end she tells her mother that she's got to mend things with her mother, I mean the grandmother really, but that's at the end of everything, and the mother comes out in the garden of this house where they live, her daughter and her husband who no one's ever met, though they've been married for years it must be, her daughter's nearly leaving school, and she brings out some drinks, the daughter I mean, I really, really want to go to the South of France, it looked beautiful, and then first she says, Who's this mother to her mother and the daughter, I mean the grown-up woman, the mother of the girl says nothing, but her mother who's wearing still the old coat that she was at the beginning of the movie, she says, I am only a visitor, my dear, or something like that, and then the husband takes a look at her and –

The builder had poured a measured tablespoonful of oil into a frying pan, and now turned the heat on underneath it. The builder's wife could not stand it any longer.

Is there much more of this, she said to the builder's daughter.

Oh, it was fantastic, the builder's daughter said. More of what, what do you mean. I wish I could remember what it was called.

Has anyone ever told you that telling the plots of films, it's really boring, the builder's wife said.

That's not very nice, the builder said.

It's just so bloody boring, the builder's wife said. Every day's exactly the same round here. Nothing ever happens. You could wipe out Tuesday and Wednesday would be exactly the same. You could repeat Wednesday before Thursday came and nobody would ever notice. The least you can do is not to be so bloody boring.

Well, I'll spare myself the trouble next time, the builder's daughter said.

It sounded like something somebody would say before leaving, but the builder's daughter was no good at that sort of thing: she fell silent and stayed where she was, leaning against the island cupboards and work surface. The builder continued with his methodical process. Perhaps there was something in the frown of his eyes that told you how he felt. But it was true. He was boring. The daughter was very boring. The son was boring. Maybe one day his son and his daughter would leave home – what were they doing here, in her house? There was no pressure from the ordinary way of living to make the builder leave home, however. And now the phone rang – not anyone's mobile, but the landline that nobody ever used and that never rang. She went into the hallway and answered it.

No, she said. He can't come to the phone right now.

Yes, I'll pass the message on. What's it about?

Well, I don't know how he'll be able to help, she said.

I'm sure that's right. I expect he'll remember you, I'll tell him your name.

No, that's not what I'm saying. I'm saying he can't come out. He's not allowed to. It's the law.

No, it's not for me to suggest anything. You'll just have to cope with a loose stair rod.

No, I'm sorry. It doesn't make any difference how long you've known him, he's not going to come out. I'm telling you. We're all in difficult situations.

I think it's best if I put the phone down now. I'm sorry I can't help you.

She came back into the kitchen.

Who was that, the builder said.

Someone who wanted you to go and mend their broken stair rod. Some people have no idea. How long's it going to be?

Dinner takes the length of time to prepare that dinner takes to prepare, the builder said. It is the length of a piece of string. It is the moment that fills an hour. It is what the philosophers of past history call the time a breath takes, the time filled by a lifetime. But what is life?

The builder's daughter was laughing at this. She always enjoyed his venture into the mood of a Chinese philosopher; he had been doing it since they were small children, and addicted to a TV serial about Chinese monks who could kill with a single blow to the throat while talking about the wind under a butterfly's wings.

Fine, the builder's wife said, and left the room. One of these days she would say the wrong thing to him, rather than to some old man who claimed to be a customer, or one of his children, and the marriage would be over, but not today.

12

The father was at the top of the house. The house was a cream-coloured stone. It was three storeys high, surrounded by a garden and a driveway. On the ground floor were a sitting room, kitchen and dining room; the first floor held two bedrooms and a bedroom-cum-library; the second floor, which had once had three small bedrooms, was now given over to the father's pleasant hobbies. He went up to the second floor quite soon after breakfast each day, and worked on one of his activities. It was as cosy and enclosed as a shed. The mother spent her days downstairs in the sitting room, her nights in the bedroom on the first floor. It had been many years since she had climbed the last staircase to the second floor. It was the father's territory.

One room on the top floor was narrow under a pointed ceiling. The ceiling had two windows set in it, flush with the roof. The father had designated this room, with its large ceiling windows and full clear light, his painting room. An easel stood in the centre, and on the table by the painting chair, boxes of watercolours, a folder of paper, pencils and pastels, a jar holding brushes of different sizes and a jam jar, stained with old paint and half filled with water. The carpet underneath was old, and covered with accidents of paint. That was nobody's concern.

The larger of the other rooms was used for storage of equipment, books, and the products of the father's hobbies: folders of watercolours labelled with dates, and also models of boats, buildings and trains that had been made over the years. This room had once been the son's bedroom, but the bed and a shower in the corner of the room had long ago been removed. Now the objects and the products and the collections piled up against the William Morris wallpaper the son had chosen decades ago, and a desk that had once stood downstairs, a swivelling chair that had had its place in the library.

The father sat in the third room, holding a magnifying glass and a fine paintbrush. He was writing a word on the side of a miniature train carriage in gold paint. The third room was filled with a constructed world, a circular line of narrow rails, four or five wide. There were a dozen trains on the rails, each of which had been made by the father over forty years, cutting and shaping sheets of metal, attaching tiny shapes one to another, painting until an exact replica of a particular train from the 1930s was achieved, and the time came to start work on another. The trains, when they ran, went through the model of a town, also evoking the 1930s. Shop windows held miniature goods; pubs carried signs; a two-inch horse stood with for-ever patience in front of a brewer's cart; a barber's pole drew attention to an interior in which a tiny customer sat, his face covered with hard foam, waiting. In the windows of some of the houses interiors could be glimpsed, and parts of families. A crocodile of children walked towards the school. The businesses were neatly identified, and each was named after a member of the father's family, the son, the daughter, the grandchildren, the mother.

The father was painting a word on the side of one of the new set of carriages – not a family name, but the correct word that the carriage of this date would have borne. The last time the son had been there, he had come up to the railway room and looked around, apparently with interest, although of course he knew nothing about trains or the 1930s. He had suggested that the town the father had built was very respectable and orderly, even the pub and the police station. He had suggested, how seriously the father didn't know, that the father should turn one of the houses by the station into a brothel, fill the pavement outside the pub with drunken brawlers, construct a bank robbery, the armed robbers fleeing with sacks spilling notes, kidnappings, heroin addicts dying in back alleys, men meeting in the bushes on the other side of the bridge – bushes constructed out of torn and dyed sponge, very convincing – and the little figures in the copses having sex with each other. But the father had not done any of this, and the model town went on its own orderly way, the decade of the father's own birth. He might have a vicar going into the pub or a bookmaker's.

A voice was coming from the sitting room, two floors down. It had been calling his name for a few minutes now. He had been concentrating on the job at hand, the tiny brush and the nail-varnish-sized bottle of gold paint. Sometimes the mother called out for no good reason; wanted to share that she liked one of the paintings on the wall she was facing. Sometimes she needed a glass of water or the toilet, however. He let the calls go on for a few minutes, in general, before going down.

On the back of the door into the railway room a cork board was pinned with family photographs. Among these was a photograph of the mother before his fiftieth birthday party, thirty-five years before. She had had her hair done, and it was a vivid ginger, just as when she was a girl; she was raising a pre-party glass; she was wearing that glamorous midnight-blue long dress she used to wear to parties; she was smiling with a degree of pride at what she had done, and the table behind her was packed with dishes she had made. The food at that party had been delicious. He could have eaten it now, very happily. And fifty people had come and the son, or perhaps the daughter, had made a speech, though they were both very young, students, both of them. What a success that had been and now there would never be any more successes of that sort, unless you counted his funeral, which he wouldn't, he didn't think.

The calls were still continuing. He put down the brush and stood up. Things changed. A swimming enveloped him. The room moved. It was quiet up there, but something thumped like the stereo in a passing car. It could be his heart. This is it, he thought. But he had thought that many times before. It was very important that he get himself downstairs, where he could be found if things got worse. He got himself to his feet, and pulled himself through the door, the palm of his hand to the wall. The swimming continued and a wave of heat. When it disappeared, and he had got himself to the first floor, he should probably call for some help. That was what doctors were there for. From downstairs the sound of his name came, more emphatically, even impatiently, but there was nothing to be done for the moment.

Now he was at the top of the stairs, and with his hand on the banister he walked down. He had gone six or seven steps when the carpet beneath his feet slipped, taking him with it. The stair rod, he said as he fell, the stair rod, and the conversation he had had with that bloody woman came to his mind in outraged summary.

He sat down on the floor and his head rested against the cool metal support under the model railway. Then he opened his eyes and that was not where he was. He was on the stairs and his face was against the coarse and hot texture of the carpet. The flood of hot and the warm swimming substance that now surrounded him swelled, inflated, swallowed him. He felt as if he should spring to his feet, walk forward and in a moment he would be free of the sensation, like leaving a room. There was some pain somewhere nearby and a voice making small noises that must be his own. The sounds around grew

remote and tinny, a voice calling from downstairs, the whis-
tling screams of starlings and the rattle of a magpie in a tree, a
van ticking down the road. In the blanket of hot numbness
distancing him from everything he could see or hear or feel he
lay unmoving and yet plummeting. The metal support was
cold against his forehead. No, it was the carpet against his
head. His forehead was pouring with sweat.

This is it.

This is it.

This is it.

The telephone extension was at the top of the stairs, a few
steps away. If he could reach it, then he could make a phone
call. He could press a single button and call his son, or another
to summon the most helpful of the neighbours, five houses
away. The best thing to do might be to call the neighbour. She
had a key to the house. With relief he remembered that in his
pocket there was also a telephone, a mobile. The stairs moved.
The air thickened. A hot thunder struck again, and again, a
voice still calling out far away.

13

The son was making Molotoff pudding in the kitchen. He
believed it was originally Malakoff, conflated with the rioter's
Molotoff cocktail by some vague Portuguese cake-maker. It was
very simple, just twelve egg whites whisked into stiffness with
caramel, and baked in a ring mould. With the twelve egg yolks,
the man was planning to make a pint of mayonnaise and
enough zabaglione to stun a regiment. That morning, since
returning from the walk on which they had seen Marianne's
building on fire, he had watered the garden and, for two hours,
read *The Anatomy of Melancholy*. Now, knocking the half-filled

ring mould hard on the surface, he repeated a phrase he had read an hour before, which had given him delight. I shall place the pudding before you, husband, he said, in cod seventeenth-century, his voice lowered, and you shall gaze upon it in awe and pleasure, and raise your eyes to my face, and you shall fall upon me like a pig on pie. A pig on pie. He repeated the phrase that had almost made him yelp, and banged the ring mould again on the hard surface, to dislodge bubbles.

The phone rang again. He looked at the screen. This time he had better answer it. It was his sister who was calling.

Hello, he said. How are you?

Fine, she said. Listen. I've just had a call from their neighbour. Mum and Dad, their neighbour. What's happened. My dad called her saying he wasn't feeling well. She went round and called an ambulance. She's got a key.

What happened?

He'd collapsed. Felt very dizzy. Might have a fever. Fainted. He's gone into hospital.

Oh, Christ. It's not Covid, is it?

Of course it's not Covid.

Okay.

He might get checked over and sent home or they might have to keep him in for a while. You're going to need to go up there straight away. The neighbour's sitting with her for the moment – she saw my dad into the ambulance, then phoned me. Did she phone you?

Was it Lucy?

Was who Lucy? The woman next door? Something like that.

I'll throw some things into a bag and I'll be up there by six. I'll get a train.

You need to be up there as soon as possible.

Six is as soon as possible, the son said. He ended the call and placed the telephone on the kitchen work surface.

Pour me a drink, he said to his husband, who was in the door of the kitchen, looking at him with a question on his face.

It's only two o'clock, the husband said. What are you making? And who was that?

Molotoff pudding. Take it out of the oven in an hour and let it cool. I'll be gone by then. That – he pointed at the phone – was my sister.

Oh, Christ, what now.

My dad's fainted or something at home and they've taken him into hospital. I'm sure he's fine. But my mum's going to be on her own till he comes out.

You can't go up. It's not allowed. And it's not safe, going to St Pancras and getting a train. What happens if –

I know what happens if. Don't really have a choice. It's fine, the son said. I don't mind a few days with my mum. I'll be super-careful, wear gloves and everything.

I'll come with you.

No, you won't, the son said. You stay here. Look at that Molotoff pudding I've just made that needs eating. I'm not throwing twelve eggs away.

Because the previous week the supermarkets had been stripped bare of eggs. They had gone from one shop to another, from the gentleman butcher where a chicken cost twenty pounds, right down even to the strip-lit convenience store with its shelves of super-strength cider for street drinking; everyone had shrugged when appealed to, like characters in bad novels, shrugging and shrugging, and one even sighing, everyone had said, once they had finished their stock gestures, that it couldn't be helped. But yesterday the son had gone to the supermarket, had queued with his shopping basket and had come across a single pile of egg cartons. He had bought twenty-four, in triumph; the wasteful construction of an extravagant pudding was a gesture of defiance.

I see your point, the husband said seriously.

It's not a problem, the son said. I'll put my students off till next week. Oh, Christ, that seminar. Oh, fuck.

Just stop it, the husband said, laughing.

14

Angela didn't care who knew it – she was being driven round the bend, living with Bev full time. Doolally, barmy, bonkers. What a lot of lovely words. But you've been living with the silly cow for ten years, Katy had said. True enough, but when you worked it out, you were at work or going to work or getting ready for work or doing some work at home for five days a week minimum, more like six realistically. So, in fact, thanks to the law, you only saw the silly cow for about twelve hours a week. Only when you were stupid enough to go away on holiday –

Don't remind me, Katy said. That villa in Tuscany.

Quite, Angela said.

This was like an unending version of the villa in Tuscany, with tears and thrown plates and home truths served up over breakfast. Bev was bored and back on the white stuff. Lockdown and the end of international travel didn't appear to have affected the business of the drug-dealers of London, one of whom (Darren) showed up every Friday afternoon, prompt as a press conference, or prompter. Angela wished she didn't know his name.

I suppose Marriage Guidance accepts lesbians, Katy said.

On Zoom, Angela said. Apparently. I can't face that.

Well, maybe this is one of those rough patches every marriage goes through, Katy said, rattling it off rather. Then Zoom told them they'd had their forty-five minutes. They called it a day.

Frankly, Angela didn't know what she'd do without Uncumber. You could always justify leaving the house by just shouting. Cumby wants a walk, up the stairs. Good old Uncumber – she almost always went along with it. She was five, a miniature Schnauzer, lavishly bearded and fiercely eyebrowed; she loved Angela beyond reason.

They were in the park, and into the long avenue of plane trees, when Uncumber trotted off to greet someone she knew. She was an immensely gracious and polite dog; her passionate enthusiasm only showed in the mad metronome of her tail. The dog she was greeting was a familiar one, a gingerish terrier of sorts. Sometimes you got to know the names of dogs in the park and their owners only as 'Bobby's owner'. This one, though, was Brutus and his owner was Natasha. She'd introduced herself properly; a handsome large woman with broad, almost Slavic cheekbones – was it her ridiculous name that made you think that? And a flood of blonde-streaked hair, hardly attended to. She had a kid, maybe two, a surprising way of yawning noisily without restraint or apology, and a husband who was an accountant.

I thought that was Uncumber, she said. Bless her. Bearing up?

Well enough, considering the first thing my wife said to me this morning.

Go on, Natasha said.

You're such a cunt, Angela said. She meant it, too.

What had you done?

Opened the curtains, Angela said. But it could have been anything at all.

It's such a nightmare, Natasha said. What goes on behind closed doors.

She's not hitting me, Angela said. I'd tell you if she was. I'd tell someone.

Oh, you must, Natasha said, but somehow lightly, as if in a moment she would walk away with Brutus's eager little trot at her side and never think of Angela again. Something of that must have shown in Angela's face, because against all regulations, Natasha stepped forward; she embraced Angela. For a few moments Angela's face was against Natasha's; she felt half buried in a fall of thick blonde hair, smelling rather deliciously of apple and mint, a supermarket shampoo, but wonderful all the same. Natasha said goodbye apologetically; a world rose up where husbands, wives, children, and the Law were abolished, where two calm women with their dogs walked down a long dappled avenue of plane trees, returning to the house they lived in, with love. It was, in fact, half past ten. There was a meeting at twelve to prepare for; that SenStar business.

15

The son had never truly lived in the house. The mother had always wanted to live in a Victorian house with gables and bays, a cellar and a servants' attic; the father had always wanted a house big enough to find a space for a full-scale model of a railway. They had finally moved into this house nearly forty years before, the same month that the son had left home to go to university. Now the son sat with the mother and told her the story of their four houses.

This isn't my house, the mother said. I don't know when we're going home.

This is your house, the son said. You love your house, I know.

It's not my house, the mother said.

The first house you lived in, the son said, after you married, was in Cromwell Avenue, a little house but very nice. I was born in that house, do you remember? And you didn't have a phone, and it was a very cold and snowy February, so my dad had to put his wellies on and go to the end of the road to phone the midwife. And by the time she got there I was almost born. And then you moved to the house in Malden Road, with a long garden, with fruit trees at the end, and Mr and Mrs Griffiths living next door …

He went on, everything that he could remember: the memory of before school, returning from walking his sister to school and his mother standing and talking to a friend for ever in the cold and, bafflingly, the dark, somewhere above him. (Years later he read about the government in the 1960s experimenting and abandoning Summer Time: it really had been dark in the morning.) As he went on, the look in his mother's eyes sharpened and brightened, lost that dull underwater confused thickened layer. She remembered. He carried on, and when he got to the little story of how they had chosen and moved into the house they were in, everything had clarified, brightened, become certain.

Would you like a cup of tea? the son said, when he had finished.

I've always loved reading, the mother said, opening the book on her lap. I've read this one before, I know. But you can always read a good book more than once.

We'll have some tea, the son said. Won't be a tick.

The son had never lived permanently in this house, and the organization of the kitchen was opaque to him; there were dinner plates in three separate cupboards; the coffee was kept in the spice cupboard and the tea in the glasses cabinet. There were biscuits, but the plain ones were kept in a barrel on the work surface, the chocolate ones in an ancient box that a supermarket had once sold biscuits for cheese in, on top of the freezer in the pantry. It had taken some time to get on top of all this, which made perfect sense to the father and, once, the mother. The milk, thankfully, was in the fridge.

These few days would be an unusual, static, forgettable interlude. There was nothing to do and no action to take. He had arrived three days before. His mother had looked up from her conversation with the neighbour when he walked into the room; her expression was incredulously joyful. Since then, he had cooked for her, sat and talked to her, walked with her round the garden, and reassured her at regular intervals that although the father was ill in hospital he would be home soon. She accepted this; in half an hour she would ask again. You were not allowed to visit the father in hospital. Twice a day he phoned the ward, and a nurse would explain that everything was going well, that there was no cause for concern, but the father would not be discharged just yet. The son didn't mind. The interlude extended. It had no events and nothing that happened had any consequences. It was as far from the dynamic exercise of consequence as could be imagined; not *This happened and as a result this happened*. Rather, *This happened; this was said; then it happened again; it was said again; and nobody minded*. In a moment he would go back into the sitting room and his mother would say that she had always loved reading, and he would agree, that he, too, loved reading, and they would drink a cup of tea together.

In the kitchen the telephone sounded; the penetrating summons of the SMS bell. It was either his husband or his sister; he looked and it was his sister.

Call me between 12.20 and 12.30 later today the message said. He went on making the cups of tea. He took them through to the sitting room, and they sat for a while, talking about things to hand. The strident call tone could be heard from the kitchen from time to time: three more messages of increasing purposefulness, it proved.

Will do, the son texted back. Almost immediately the phone rang.

I can talk now but briefly, the daughter said.

No trouble, the son said.

What's going on, the daughter said.

Everything seems fine at the hospital, the son said. We're just having a cup of tea and reading our books.

This sort of situation can't go on, the daughter said. He's going to have to put her in a home. I've been phoning round care homes and I've got a list that you need to look at and research.

This is a new development, the son said, and was quite quickly made aware that he had failed to keep the sarcastic tone from his voice.

After a few minutes the daughter said, Just fucking do it.

I'm not going to fucking do it, the son said, and hung up.

The phone rang again and the son ignored it. A moment later a text message arrived. The son read it, and sent a message back: *I very much hope that when you speak to my dad in hospital, you don't take this tone with him.*

Fuck off.

When the son tried to send a message back – *Honestly? Not very helpful* – he found that he had been blocked from communicating with his sister.

When the son's husband phoned later in the morning, the son retold the conversation, with some ornamentations. The son's husband recognized the ornamentations for what they were, and laughed at the telling.

Simplifies things, the son said.

I'm not sure that's something that can be simplified for ever, the son's husband said.

16

Once, a friend of the son's, a novelist, had said to him that the relationship between a brother and a sister was completely mysterious to him. The friend had been an only child. The son had smiled as if in possession of some secret and arcane knowledge, but afterwards had thought of what he might have said: me too, me too.

Fuck off, and then blocked. Could that happen? It had happened. Exotic relationships, covered by siblinghood, crowded in on him. One friend had a brother who was a recovering heroin addict, living in the remote countryside. When brought to London, the brother had been timid and wide-eyed. After a silent hour in company, he had said to one of his brother's friends, Are you all doctors, then? Another friend had barely talked to his brother in decades. Their mother died; a burden lifted; they started to talk at the funeral; they totted things up; the brother had six children with different women, some infants, others long-estranged young adults. Another friend, a woman of nearly eighty, was met by chance with two sisters, one the friend's twin, all shopping for food in an Oxford Street department store. Before he said hello, he heard his friend say something from the nursery, three-quarters of a century before. You're both being horrid, she said. I hate you. I hate you. I hate you, the twin said with emphasis. They were all grandmothers; one was walking with a stick, but their basket was full of little treats, and they hated each other, they comfortably said.

Once the son had thrown an orange at the daughter, and had broken her glasses.

Once he had sat with her on a bench in Fitzrovia and let her cry for an hour because her boyfriend had left her.

Once she had said to him, I know what you said to that boy at the party and I've told Mum and Dad so they'll know what sort of person you are, and he had said, What, that I'm gay?

Once he had taken a bulb out of a lamp when it was still plugged in and stuck his finger into the socket and then, impressed by the sensation, had told the daughter to do the same and was astonished when she screamed and ran to Mummy.

Once she had told him that she would be moving into a flatshare in Kilburn and then two days later that she would not, because the girl whose flat it was had turned out to be a lesbian who had sexually assaulted her before she had unpacked her suitcases.

Once they had gone together to a school disco and she had broken off from snogging a boy to tell him that a group of fifth-formers were taking the piss out of how he was standing.

Once they had gone to Paris together for four days and had eaten every night in terrible restaurants from a book called *Paris for Paupers* and on the way home had talked about which of the meals had been a waste.

Once she had got married and he had had nothing to do, and had been placed on the table between her boss's wife and her new husband's Australian cousin in the middle of a European tour.

Once he had had a Christian phase and she had sent him a birthday card wishing him the love of our Lord Jesus Christ because she thought it was funny and would upset him.

Once he had suggested that she buy a green woollen dress, because he thought it suited her, and she wore it to her first job out of university, once, before her supervisor told her it wasn't appropriate for the office.

Once she had spent an afternoon washing her hair and tying it in tiny plaits to produce the effect of frizz, a twenty-four-hour perm, and he had watched the whole process, fascinated.

Once he had cycled to the hospital where she had just had her first baby, and found the mother and father by the bedside, pink and delighted.

Once she had insisted that he take her elder child abroad for a birthday present, then three years later her younger child, two trips that remained in the son's mind years later as experiences of horror, vacuity, shame and ludicrous expense; the sight of a resentful adolescent kicking a stone in a Roman piazza and announcing that he was going back to the hotel because he was bored.

Once she had played the guitar on a studio LP made by their school, her name printed on the back as one of the soloists on track six, 'Spanish Melody', and it had seemed miraculous to the son.

Once, years after it had stopped being necessary to watch expenditure closely, the son was in Paris on holiday. It was an absurd holiday, an anti-honeymoon, though there would be a honeymoon after the wedding as well as a holiday before. He went with the man he was about to marry to one of the restaurants they had found in *Paris for Paupers*. It was called Chartier. It was a huge hall, brown and silver and brilliant with hard lighting and hard surfaces, crowded with tables, hard-faced waiters pushing between chairs, huge trays above their shoulders. The noise and echoes of raised voices were immense, and the glitter of the mirrors and the glass-cased desserts and crudités. Wow, the husband or rather at that point fiancé said, as they were unsmilingly seated, handed a tattered menu. This is extraordinary. I came here with my sister, the son said. I was eighteen. She said afterwards it had been a waste of a dinner. It looks really good, the husband said. They ordered. The crudités came in seconds, and were wonderful, a crisp bite of herbal celeriac in an eggy coat of mayonnaise; the red wine was sour and perfect and the stuff of laughter, romance, a couple about to marry. This is ridiculous, the husband said. I love it. His eyes were shining.

At the next table five Australians were arguing over their bill with an impatient waiter. I wish I was still a carnivore, the husband said, as the bavette came; he reached out and took a chip. My sister hated it, the son said. She said it was all a bit of a rip-off. She said the same thing the one time she went to India, the husband said. I don't know how the whole country could be a rip-off. It's a terrible rip-off, the son said, getting you to spend your money, and what do you get for it in the end? Some mouldy old Mughal miniature, just some awful court portrait, what a rip-off, hundreds of years old, never falling for that one again. You do like it, though, the husband said, laughter in his eyes, because that had been the husband's birthday present, a week earlier. I love it, the husband said, but that's because I'm an idiot that the rip-off merchants just see coming, every, every time. I wish I'd had the steak, the husband said, it looks so good, apart from the blood.

And then once the father had said to the son what the daughter had told him, and he had sent her an angry message saying that she shouldn't speak to anyone as she had spoken to their father.

Once she had responded and said, Fuck off, and then blocked her brother from communicating with her again.

Maybe that only happened once, like all the other events that only happened once, like everything. And all of those events were causes of other events, and led to conclusions that concluded nothing, but only caused further events, and so on.

17

And then there are other events, other chains of causality, and they might run something like this:

17.1 A couple have a child, a daughter.

17.2 The daughter is bright, but on the morning of one of her A-level exams, she suffers from a blinding headache and cannot write what she undoubtedly knows.

17.3 The daughter's A-level results are in line with predictions, apart from one subject, which falls short of the grade required by her first-choice university.

17.4 At her second-choice university, this woman is filled with rage and dissatisfaction.

17.5 She meets and quickly leaves one man after another, studying the same sort of subjects as she is. They strike her as pathetic.

17.6 She is determined to be a success in life, professionally speaking.

17.7 And yet not to be mired in a relationship with someone who may be more successful than her, or slightly less successful.

17.8 Her parents die within two years of each other: at twenty-five, she has a house of her own.

17.9 After three years, she decides to make the house her own.

17.10 She employs a builder to make some changes; he is recently divorced and has two small children.

17.11 She marries him.

17.12 After ten years, an epidemic strikes. She continues to work; he is placed on furlough.

17.13 Prolonged exposure in the house leads her to realize she does not care for his children at all, and not much for him, the dissatisfaction rooted in her from who knows what causes lighting her up like a shop-window display.

17.14 Answering the phone, she dismisses, impatiently, a customer who wants a small but important job done.

17.15 The customer's house goes on containing a danger.

17.16 The customer falls and is placed in hospital.

17.17 Because the customer's wife needs to be supported, the customer's son travels up on the train, against regulations.

17.18 The customer is released from hospital.

17.19 The customer's son travels back on the train, at a time when more people are physically close to him than is permitted or advisable.

17.20 Another cause approaches, from another direction, an event-chain of strangers, linking hands and coughing.

18

Got Darren on WhatsApp, Martin said. You want anything?

Huh, Scott said. He'd just stretched out for a moment on Martin's sofa then, blam, he was asleep. Huh. What – er –

I said, Martin said, I've got Darren coming over. Do you want anything?

I'm skint, bruv, Scott said. Stick to beer.

Yeah, right, Martin said, but he wasn't bothered. Martin was loaded – German or Austrian or something, his dad had a big castle and made tractors or submarines or who gave a fuck. Martin just had a big dick and a generously hospitable nature.

He lived in an immense flat in Cadogan Square, extending over what must have been three houses. He and Scott were on the sofa in the drawing room. Scott was lying, his feet in Martin's lap. They were naked. Martin still had an erection, batting gently against the soles of Scott's bare feet. Impressive. He must have injected it or something. The windows looked out over the tops of the trees in the garden you had to live there to have a key for.

So there's that Giorgio coming over, Martin said. And he said he'd bring Tony and Andy. And Kingsley. And that Reynolds, the guy who's supposed to be a famous writer, journalist, whatever.

Oh, great, Scott said. He's built like a, he's like a fucking engine, a motor, that Reynolds.

And I think I am going to persuade the handsome Darren to stay for a little while on his own account, Martin said. I am sure he would like to.

Bullshit, Scott said.

Well, we will see, Martin said. I am just now going to fetch the rubber sheeting to protect the floor and the tarpaulins to protect the sofas and the chairs and to wash the dildos and to put some lube out and to wash my ass but not the rest, because when the boys come, I want me to smell like an animal, you know what I am saying?

Grr, Scott said. Then the buzzer went and it was Reynolds, first in line.

19

The subject had wanted to do it in person. He had told the books desk that he was too old to be messing about with – well, he had meant Zoom and Google Hangout, but who

knows what he said? 'Too old' might have meant that he
couldn't meet anyone; that he was vulnerable, as they said. But
the idea of Henry Ricks Bailey being *vulnerable* after the life
he'd led – the decades in Soho, the story about him setting his
publisher's offices on fire, the one about him trying to sell that
poet Susan Liddell in a camel market on a British Council trip
to Mali, or was it in a fishmonger's in Oslo? – that was hard to
take seriously. He had a book out, but when did he not have a
book out? The word from the books desk was that he was in a
mood to talk about Sophie, sixty years dead now; a suicide at
twenty-six, leaving three perfect tiny novels and a grave in
Highgate perpetually foaming with a mountain of white flowers. That second book: *White Flowers, Black Rain*. He was
going to talk about the way she had been found, darkly turgid
with blood, bloated, almost inflated, and nudging the pillars of
Vauxhall Bridge. She had thrown herself in a mile upstream. A
neat typed manuscript on her desk. That was the winter of
1962; a bleak winter all round for those who could remember
it. Sophie had known what Henry was capable of doing, and
had posted a carbon copy of that last novel to her sister with
clear instructions. But he had not destroyed it, or tried to; it
had been published exactly, word for word, as she had left it,
and that heartbreaker would live for ever. *The Fire in Winter*.
Nothing Henry Ricks Bailey had done would last half as long.

And now Reynolds was in the conservatory of the house in
Rickmansworth. A good two hours' journey from Reynolds's
flat in Clapham, a strange journey in empty, rattling trains, that
unfamiliar purple line with its pre-war air taking him deep into
what looked like the country. A taxi had taken him to the old
rectory, stately in a sea of gravel – of course he had still been
married to that first wife when she threw herself into the river.
The royalties of *The Fire in Winter* would be his until it fell out
of copyright in twelve years' time. The fifth wife had come to

the front door, masked. A thin woman, a lilac cardigan over her shoulders, her blue eyes large and knowledgeable; streaks of grey in her smooth blonde hair. He had married her when she was twenty-five; now she must be forty. She had told him briefly to walk round the side of the house. He had come in through the open door to the conservatory. Two chairs faced each other, fifteen feet apart. Reynolds placed his phone on the table in front of one, and pressed record; he could hear the steps of the approaching Henry Ricks Bailey. He sat in the other. He waited.

Don't shake his hand, a female voice called.

Of course I fucking won't, Henry Ricks Bailey said. He came into the room. He was old; the impression was powerful, from the immediate embrocation smell to the hands clutched into claws. His neat white shirt had been bought for a larger person; his grey and wrinkled neck sat within the fastened collar like a single gladiolus stalk in a vase. He fixed Reynolds with a red-rimmed eye that could have come from crying. It's you, then, Henry Ricks Bailey said.

Yes, it's me, Reynolds said. I'm from the paper. I'm here to talk to you about the new book.

I know why you're here, Henry Ricks Bailey said, sitting down in the well-padded garden chair, businesslike and brisk in his movements. I wasn't expecting them to send you again. You interviewed me when I won that book prize. Double-page spread and you said I had surprised people who had written me off years before.

I don't think that was me, Reynolds said. He had read the profile on the train. It had been written by Victoria Winton in short order when Henry Ricks Bailey had won his big prize; to the practised eye, it was apparent that Winton had never read any of Henry Ricks Bailey's novels ('*The Urchin in Autumn* reduced me to tears with its delicacy and underlying power') and he wondered how the interview had gone.

It was definitely you, Henry Ricks Bailey said. I expect you interview so many people it's hard to remember. In fact I think you were wearing the same shoes that you have on now. So. What are we here for.

The new novel, Reynolds said, and paused. There was a difficulty here that he hoped Henry Ricks Bailey would solve.

Ah, yes, Henry Ricks Bailey said.

Why the title, Reynolds said.

The title, Henry Ricks Bailey said. An expectant silence came between them, and Henry Ricks Bailey's interrogation of a look. There seemed to be no way out of it.

A Symphony by Sibelius, Reynolds said.

Sibelius, Henry Ricks Bailey said lightly, correcting him.

I wondered why that was so important, Reynolds said.

Why what was, Henry Ricks Bailey said. Christ.

The symphony, Reynolds said. It comes up once. When the hero goes to the concert on his own.

Henry Ricks Bailey looked him over; he turned his head towards the conservatory door. Somewhere near at hand a dishwasher was being loaded.

Let's drop this terrible crap, Henry Ricks Bailey said. I know what the rules are. You pretend to be interested in my writing. I get softened up with your fervent admiration. Then you ask me about a wife I used to be married to, decades ago.

That's not quite fair, Reynolds said. I loved this novel. It's about such an important issue.

What is that important issue, Henry Ricks Bailey said. In your view.

This old fool had made up his mind to be as disagreeable as possible, but there was no reason for Reynolds to respond in the same way. He would get his chance in print, looking at the wrinkled old fool and his enraged red stare. Henry Ricks Bailey sits in his conservatory, comfortable in the beautiful Swedish ashwood garden chair with sage upholstery; it was paid for by the writing of a wife he'd driven to suicide. Perhaps paid for in part.

I don't think many writers have written about the effect it has on your old age, the decision not to have children.

Do you have children?

No.

Neither do I. So I don't suppose the issue, as you describe it, needs exploring. You'll find out. Or not.

Reynolds waited. The red light on his mobile phone went on shining, indicating that the conversation, such as it was, was being recorded.

How has the lockdown affected your writing, Reynolds said. Your ability to write. Some people have found it a very inspiring situation.

I was thinking about Evelyn Waugh the other day, Henry Ricks Bailey said. An apparently intelligent and charming woman met him at a party, and talked to him very civilly about how much she admired his books. She said, among other things, that he was the most elegant prose stylist she had ever read. Waugh went away. Forgive me if I told you this story the last time you interviewed me.

No, no.

Waugh went away. The next day a country neighbour called on him, a very old friend. When she heard about this conversation, she said, I hope you weren't too horrible to her. Waugh's tone, telling the story, had been dangerously close to laughter. Oh, no, Waugh said. I wasn't horrible to her. I was merely amused at the idea the poor beast knows one prose style from another.

I see, Reynolds said.

Now why was I telling that story, Henry Ricks Bailey said.

I think you were probably aiming at being rude to me, Reynolds said, giving up.

It is interesting to me, Henry Ricks Bailey went on tranquilly. When people talk about novels, if they talk at all, they talk about the subject of those novels. Or they talk about the life of the person who wrote it. This is a wonderful book, they say. It's about a couple who fall in love during the Rwandan genocide, they say. Or You must read this book. It's by this woman who came to England as a refugee but her husband beat her. It's as if all one had to do to write a novel is pick up a big box of stuff in one room and move it into the next.

The intractable struggle with words and meaning, Reynolds said, pleased to supply a comment.

Very good. I don't suppose anyone much reads novels any more, Henry Ricks Bailey said. Someone who does looks at things differently. When you write a novel, you think about causes. And you think about consequences. I write a chapter; I ask myself what will follow from what I wrote; something happens. Helen Schlegel takes Leonard Bast's umbrella by mistake; he retrieves it; they hand over their card; his mistress confronts them; they take an interest; they lose him his job. And so on, until the machinery of the novel, or life and its consequences, kills him under a falling bookshelf. Take your pick. In life, things follow one another. Even out of this absurd and artificial encounter, something will result.

I will write about it, Reynolds said.

And my publicist will phone your editor and abuse him, Henry Ricks Bailey said.

Your novels are beautifully constructed, Reynolds said.

My novels are beautifully written, Henry Ricks Bailey said, with a small ballet of the hands, a gesture of disappointment. Don't forget *beautifully written*. Poor beast. I don't know about beautifully constructed. It might be just noticing things. One small thing happens out of nowhere; something else happens;

another thing, and another, and at the end of the chain, the world ends.

Inevitably, Reynolds said. He had no idea how he was going to get Henry Ricks Bailey back to the point. This stuff would not do for readers of the magazine on a Saturday morning.

A moral point, Henry Ricks Bailey said. If fiction has made you wonder what follows on from *this*, for *him*, for *her*, you are thinking about other people. Through other people's eyes. If you think about whether you should write *I am walking from Whitstable to Ramsgate* or *Every Monday he walked from Whitstable to Ramsgate* then … then I don't know what will follow for you. I don't know how people manage otherwise. Do you know the other thing that everyone always asks? How much of this is real?

Why Whitstable, why Ramsgate? Reynolds said.

Henry Ricks Bailey looked at him. His expression was of sadness, even despair.

That's not worth going into, he said. Subject matter. Whitstable is subject matter.

You've lost me, Reynolds said finally.

I thought I might have, Henry Ricks Bailey said.

Consequences is an interesting word, Reynolds said, ploughing on. I wonder – you've never really talked about the day Sophie Anstruther killed herself. It's many years ago now. Do you think the time may have come –

Some time ago, the noises in the kitchen had come to an end. Behind Henry Ricks Bailey, in the dark hall leading from the conservatory into the house, a slight figure stood. Henry Ricks Bailey's fifth wife, the marriage that had succeeded, paused between two ceiling-high bookcases, listening. She was not hiding herself. Would she intervene? It would make a good piece, the story of how he was thrown out of prizewinning novelist Henry Ricks Bailey's house for asking uncomfortable questions.

Do you think the time may have come for you to set the record straight, Reynolds said.

Oh, setting the record straight, Henry Ricks Bailey said. That you could ever do such a thing. This is called life, you know, and there are only points of view. Well. Let me try to remember.

Two hours later, Reynolds was on a Northern Line Underground train (Bank branch) heading back to Clapham Common. It was unexpectedly quite crowded. In his head were the first few sentences of the piece he was going to write. An excitement like the first itches of a fever tingled at his mouth. What Henry Ricks Bailey had said to him. The things Henry Ricks Bailey had said. The train jolted. Reynolds had to grab hold of the upright yellow pole.

20

At St Pancras the son had thought about getting an Uber. But the app was directing him to a point half a mile away for a pick-up. The Underground would do perfectly well. The Northern Line (Bank branch) would take him all the way home. There were not many people waiting on the platform, but in the first three or four stops, the carriage filled. A woman sat down in the seat next to him. Without making a point, he got up. You never knew. He would risk causing offence. He stood facing the doors. To keep his balance he took hold of the upright yellow pole. In less than an hour he would be coming through his front door. His husband would be there. He would give him a kiss. Then they would probably sit down and have their dinner in front of the television. Everything else could wait.

THREE

THE HERO UNDERTAKES A JOURNEY AWAY FROM HIS ENVIRONMENT

The path between the houses was still secure. Quentin trusted this route to the beach between garden fences. The public roads he avoided, but the outsiders hadn't discovered the secret suburban way through. He had never considered it until recently. The suburb had been built between the wars, an estate of brick bungalows behind the pebble beach, a patchwork of once neat gardens. Crazy paving and privet, Quentin said to himself, not describing it accurately, but through association. There was no privet, but there ought to have been; jasmine still shaded the front doors, like a porch, casting out its heavy odour of ripe banana. Single apple trees sprouted from little circular beds in the middle of what, only months ago, had been neat trimmed lawns. The path between the houses must have had some purpose behind it. All he had thought about when he bought the house as a weekend retreat was that you could get up, put on your swimsuit (one of six), dressing-gown (one of three, one silk and two towelling) and one pair out of his eleven flip-flops. You could be in the sea in five minutes, like Noël Coward.

There was no way of telling whether there were people living in the bungalows since the lights had gone out. You would not draw attention to your house by lighting candles in your front room. Sometimes, from the back kitchen where he sat in the evenings, he had heard a door opening and quietly shutting, or glimpsed a flicker of light from a window three plots away. Now, during the day, the houses were silent, their doors and windows closed. The owners might have gone somewhere else; they might be inside, existing as unobtrusively as they could, living on cans and preserved vegetables in bottles. While they lasted. If they were there, they would be no more likely to make a noise moving about the house than they would be to start up the electric mower, and trim the front lawn. They might be there, and talking in whispers. Or they could be dead. When he walked between the houses, he held his breath. You did not know what you might start to smell. Oh, houses, he said to himself, knowing where he had read it as a child, houses, how I hate you.

Quentin knew that his neighbours immediately to the right were still there. Two days ago, he had seen movement through the side window that mirrored the side window on his house, eight feet away. It might have been the adult son, the one who wore feather boas and practised with his mother's makeup; that gesture had looked like Sarah Bernhardt's farewell bow, in outline. That bungalow had been number 82 Savile Crescent. Savile Crescent, running through the Savile estate. He was not sure it still made any sense to go on calling it that, or his number number 80.

The sky was white and blank and hard as a blank sheet of paper. The sun spread evenly across the thin veil of high cloud. He had passed between three pairs of bungalows, the path dog-legging it between properties. There was the back of old Raine's bungalow, the greedy widow with a poodle in a push-chair on rainy days. Raine liked singing the songs of Andrew Lloyd Webber. She kept the price of bungalows closest to her affections, next to the dog. Whenever they had met on the street, Raine walking or pushing her idle black poodle Buckley,

Quentin on his way to or from his morning swim, she had said much the same thing: I know what you paid for your house, she would say. When the time comes I'm going to sell mine and if I do as well as that with it, I'm moving to a little flat in Dover. Four hundred thousand pounds! I'm glad my father's not here to see how mad things have got.

That had been a year ago. What the houses were worth now he couldn't guess. The mortgage payments must have stopped with the end of the banks. Nobody was coming to reclaim the debt. The back of Raine's bungalow could be glimpsed, number twenty, glassy and closed in as an Alzheimer's gaze. The symbols that had appeared from nowhere on the back fences, slashed in white paint, a couple of nights ago, had made some distinction of her property: an equals sign with a diagonal line. Others bore a left-pointing arrow; Quentin's fence, and Linda's, both had a rudimentary spiral. Nobody could say what they indicated, or who had done it. Just trying to scare us, Raine said. But my dad, he went through the Blitz. I'm not scared. The last time he had seen Raine had been two weeks before, on his way to his morning swim. She had said something different from her usual comment. Don't go down to the beach on your own, she had said. The boys are out of control. They came across a stranger, an out-of-towner, didn't recognize him, a thief. Only gone and killed him, haven't they. Left him there. I'd watch it if I were you. Don't be scared, but don't you be putting yourself in the way of anything. Even a big fellow like you needs to watch it.

I'll watch it, Quentin said. He did not believe her. These were the stories that escalated and circulated without check – and who were *the boys*? The worst he had seen on the beach might have been their work. It was his walk towards dusk. A clear day. There was nobody else around. He had seen some kind of shape – a sculpture, an object, an arrangement – from the top of the escarpment, where the grass was beginning to grow on a previously smooth municipal sward. Grass was growing everywhere, as if finally untethered. He had made his way down in interest and some dread. It was a post and a cross-post, tied together with string. On it was a dead bird. It was not a wild bird, but someone's pet, a large grey parrot, its head limp and dangling. They had slashed at it with a knife; its throat was cut. The wings were spread wide and stapled to the cross beam. One of the wings was broken, perhaps before the bird had been killed. A parrot was big and confident in life; spread out and murdered like this, its little torso was pathetically small and frail. Someone had lured it; perhaps found it in an abandoned house; made a gesture of friendship with nuts and feed; had seized it in a towel or a sack. Parrots were strong intelligent birds; Quentin hoped this one had done some damage to its tormentors before they killed it. They had stamped on it, breaking a wing, and finally killed it with a knife. The poor beast had suffered. Some ritual had followed. The base of the crucifix and the pebbles beneath were blackened with fire, though it had not spread to the body of the poor parrot. Anyone who would do this would do the same to a pet dog or cat. He would not warn Raine on Buckley's behalf. They had done it to amuse themselves and perhaps to warn off strangers. They might do it again, or this might be enough for them. What he hoped for Buckley was that he might run away before Raine died, shed the shackles of his confinement as he might shed the shackle of his name, which had only ever been a means of knowing that he was wanted, or summoned. Quentin hoped when the time came Buckley would forget all that, and feast in the street on the rats he hunted.

What a fucking shithole, Quentin said to himself, with amusement or, at any rate, with something like a performance of amusement. There was no one to hear his performance. It took place in his head. One day soon he was going to break into the uninhabited houses and take the stores in the kitchen cupboards. He was all right for the moment. Ten days ago he had filled a trolley from the back of a supermarket, not quite gutted of goods. The three hundred cans of food would keep him going for a while longer. What a fucking shithole.

In London it might be worse. In Kentish Town it would be worse. He let his mind run through the blockbuster violence he would commit in defence of his house in Kentish Town, the front door lying off the hinges, the larder emptied, the Heal's furniture hacked up and burning on the polished-wood floors. In comes Quentin, biceps bared, with the single line on his lips: I've come for what's mine. There would be no more films on at the Kentish Town multiplex. It had been closed for five years now. You might as well play the epics of vengeance in your own head. He wondered where Scott was. What had happened to him, what had been done to him.

The path between the houses took a sharp turn to the right, and emerged behind a line of beach huts. This was why Quentin had wanted to buy a house here. The opening up. The sea as flat and turgid as a lake, swelling upwards flatly and barely breaking into waves on the shore. Under the shrill brightness of the thin-veiled cloud the sea was green or grey. The wooden stakes, marking the beach out into fifty-metre segments, still slid into the sea – the groynes, he remembered, a word he had only learnt after he'd bought the house. Fishing boats lay on the pebbled beach on their sides, each of them ripped open by people in search of whatever fishing boats could hold. The day was completely calm. A mile out to sea the mad ballet of the wind turbines still continued, cycling their leg in the busy air, supplying power somehow, to who and what and how no one could say. Every morning, arriving at the beach and seeing these forty mad giants revolving far away, a conversation with his confident father returned to him.

You don't think, his father said, it's the strength of the wind turning those bloody things?

This was two years ago, in a car driven by his father, out to a country pub where they would serve you quietly, so long as you sat in the garden and kept shtum, as his father said.

What's turning them, then, Quentin had said.

You think it's the wind? Ha, ha, ha. What's the government want you to think? That's the question you've always got to answer. What's the government want you to think.

Well, what does the government want me to think?

Wants you to think they've found a marvellous new source of electricity. Basically for nothing. Mind you, his father said, lighting the last of a packet of More cigarettes, they can't be allowed to stand there not moving. Or you'd see that there's no bloody electricity being generated there and we'd say, I say, powers that be, what the ruddy hell is going on here?

He pressed a button to open the window, and tossed the empty cigarette box out into the Kentish countryside.

I suppose they're being turned by other means, then, Quentin said. According to you.

Did you see that? his father said. Little runt. What a ruddy awful bit of driving. Glad when idiots like that are confined to quarters by the government's rules. That's another thing they want you to think. Cut me up like that, would you. What was I saying.

Wind turbines, Quentin said. He had heard all this before. Turning.

You know how they do it, his father said, closing the window.

Quentin could have given the answer his father wanted, could have said, They use electricity to turn the turbines when the wind's not blowing hard enough. But he did not.

You see, his father said, they turn a switch and the turbines are made to revolve. A little electric motor sending them revolving. It would make you laugh if it wasn't such a waste. Generate electricity when it's occasionally blowy enough. Use the electricity to turn the turbines when it's not. You know it takes Beaufort 5 to work at all. And if it gets up to Beaufort 9 it has to shut down, too strong. Bloke who knows told me. What do you think of that. Expect you and your friends talk about nothing but climate change, up there in North London.

That was the way the conversation had gone. He had wished his father would shut up then and he wished he could hear his father going on in just such a way now.

This morning he came through the gap between the beach huts onto the shingle and a man was there. He had not been so close to a stranger for weeks. At the hissing rustle of the shingle, the man turned. He was fifty, and the way he looked was not the way he was. His clothes were blackened, torn and frayed, but he was wearing a tie and his shirt was tucked into his trousers. Someone had made an attempt to cut his hair; it hovered unevenly around his ears. The pepper-and-salt beard had been excused at some point. He did not look like a man who had ever had a beard before.

Go away, the man said and that voice, too, was something he had not used until three months ago. It was the tone of someone who had already said, Go away, half a dozen times. The voice spat and cracked, a shy voice turned inside out to discover rage and fear. Go away.

I won't come close, Quentin said.

Go away, the man said again. Something was happening behind him, down at the sea's edge. Quentin fixed his look on the man's face, its rage and stricken terror, like fixing a wild animal in his gaze. He did not recognize the man. He was not a close neighbour. He had come to this beach where he did not belong.

This is our place, Quentin said. This beach, I swim here every day. Don't tell me to go away.

Go away, the man said, his voice raised. It was whipped away by the emptiness of the air between shingle and sea and sky. He had never shouted in his life, this man. Quentin looked away. Down by the water's edge, the movement he had glimpsed was a woman, a mass of clothing and a turned-up round red frightened face. That face he might have seen once before. Had she worked in a shop he'd used? Often in normal times Quentin had known that you could see a person in the same setting and know them perfectly well, and then one day glimpse the girl from the chemist's standing at the bar, the railway-station manager queuing in a bookshop, and be completely unable to place them. He might have known this woman once. What she was doing and where she now was made it impossible to say who she was or where he had ever seen her.

Oh, you filthy pigs, Quentin said. You filthy fucking pigs.

Go away, the man said. You know nothing.

This is our beach, Quentin said. This is my fucking beach. This is the place where I come out to swim in the morning. What fucking pigs you must be.

You don't know anything, the man said. What are we supposed to do. Where we live, there's nothing but the life-to-come boys. There's no running water. It'll be gone in half an hour. Three splashes of water, one big wave, and it's gone.

You filthy fucking pigs, Quentin said. I live here. This is where I live.

This is where we all live, the man said. Go away. Stop it. Stop it. Stop staring. You think she –

There was a lash-wide stare of madness to him. He would not last long. Quentin had no idea that there were places where the water had failed. The life-to-come boys – is that what he had said? These couples, they had tried different things when the water had stopped. They had dug a hole in the garden. Then they had talked it over and decided that they should come to the edge of the sea, early in the morning. No one would be around. Before, they had worked in some administrative capacity. They had solved problems. They had avoided any talk of what they would be doing. They would talk practically of what needed to be done. One would stand at the top of the beach, by the huts, while the other squatted by the sea's edge. They would finish, perhaps wash as well as they could. Then the other would come down to a place by the sea's edge, not the same place, and the other would come and stand to watch out for others. To say, Go away, to any who came. The man stared at Quentin. He was ten feet distant. He stank. How long would it be before Quentin could come down here again, in his swimsuit, his flip-flops, his towel over his shoulder and walk into the sea to swim, just at the point where the middle-aged woman was now squatting, her skirts raised around her haunches, easing her shit onto the shingle on the beach. It would be weeks; it might never happen again.

Now the woman raised her head and shouted. Go away, she said, a feeble voice without command in it. It might have been the voice of a teacher unable to keep order, but still trying to shout. Go away, she shouted, a note of pleading in her voice.

You filthy fucking pigs, Quentin said. But he turned round and went back the way he had come, between the houses. Somewhere in this was a funny story he would be able to tell to a disbelieving howling gang around a dinner table, one day. Maybe tell it to Scott. He would laugh.

There was no possibility of taking a swim that day, he said to himself. He remembered. It was twenty-five years before, and he was sitting with eleven girls and one other boy in a classroom. Each of them had a copy of the same book. This is so long, one of the girls had said, collapsing with horror. I've never read a book this long, and the other girls, one after another, had agreed. He had said nothing and the other boy had said nothing. Settle down now, please, the teacher had probably said, and in a moment they were beginning to read the novel called *Jane Eyre*, the novel set for A level. This is probably a book more for girls than for male readers, the teacher had said. He was called Mr Askwith – no, Aspinall, a tall bony sandy man, big-handed, his jointed fingers ginger-hairy and freckled when he leant over you and pointed out a sentence. Another ginger. Maybe that was where Scott started, in his mind. The teacher would probably have been Scott's age now, too. A novel that appeals to girls, Mr Askwith, no, Aspinall said again. But try your best, gentlemen. This is the first sentence, Mr Aspinall said, and read it. It isn't an important sentence, he said. But it will stay in your mind probably just because it is the first sentence of the book.

There was no possibility of taking a walk that day.

Twenty-five years later, Quentin wondered if he had remembered it correctly. There was no way of knowing. Ten years before, he had downloaded every book he thought he would ever want. He had taken the physical copies of his books to charity shops, and had the bookshelves removed, the walls behind painted white. The books were gone and life was perfected, the millions of words preserved in an infinite smallness. But now they were gone too, with the last exhaustion of the device's battery.

There was no possibility of taking a swim that day.

Something like that. He was almost home, dangling his keys.

A head rested on the top of the fence facing Quentin's back gate. It was calm in expression, as if it had waited a long time for exactly this, the appearance of Quentin from the direction of the sea.

You should keep your distance, Quentin said. Ten feet, it's supposed to be.

I haven't seen anyone for weeks apart from Mummie, Simon said. I don't see how I could possibly have caught it from anyone.

You don't know where I've been, Quentin said. I could be a danger to you.

We live next door, Simon said. You haven't been anywhere for weeks either. You just go down to the beach in the morning and come back again. Did you have a lovely swim?

I decided not to swim this morning, Quentin said.

I utterly and completely approve of that, Simon said. What a complete and utter sick-making bore that frightful swimming is. They tried to make me swim once. But I said no. I could never reconcile myself to so unnatural an activity.

Simon raised the back of his hand to his forehead. He was the son of Quentin's neighbour, Linda. He must be twenty-three, still living at home, unemployable before things changed. His unwashed hair was dyed a shining and unappetizing yellow, like a brass doorknob in the sun, his style of speech based on repeated viewings of period television dramas. In the last six months he had grown a small beard, a Vandyke pointed chin-beard. This he had not attempted to dye. He had spent his whole life in a bungalow on the coast of Kent. Why was he called Simon? Quentin thought hard, as he had thought before. Nobody under the age of fifty was called Simon; it smelt of Start-Rite shoes, the Tufty Club, tea with Mummie and the three-day week.

Mummie wants to talk to you, Simon said. You had a visitor this morning.

What do you mean? Quentin said.

A visitor, Simon said. A social call. Well, I don't know. But we heard the noise of a car engine pulling up. Mummie said,

What in the world could that be? And we rushed to the front window to see. And someone got out and went to your front door and then went back again immediately and drove off. It was the most divinely thrilling thing that has happened in the Avenue for days, weeks, months … generations. Generations.

Who was it, Quentin said.

I couldn't say, Simon said. A man.

Quentin waited. That appeared to be it. Simon went through a succession of gestures, straightening his face and hair, making a series of undecided and unconvincing noises. He had wanted to be an actor, and perhaps still did. The performance continued for a while, not acknowledging that Quentin was there, but carried out because of him.

Can I get past, Quentin said.

Of course you may, Simon said. Do you know, he went on. I am quite naked at this moment. It is my new discovery. I leave the house in the morning. I shed my outer carapace. I let the winds and breeze caress me, in the garden. It is wonderful. I am quite nude at this moment, you know, behind this fence.

No, you're not, Quentin said. Bye, Simon.

Mummie said if you were around, Simon said.

Yes, you said, Quentin said.

He went quickly by.

Quentin had been there now without a break for nine weeks. At first he had decided to stay a few days longer until things in London calmed down. The rates had been climbing and climbing, and nothing seemed to be functioning any more. For two or three weeks he had carried on working, running things through virtual meetings online. Most people, like him, had left London. The ones that had stayed were not leaving their houses, they said. One day a colleague had said that the supermarket delivery hadn't arrived; she had tried to phone, but wasn't getting any response. She supposed she could survive on the tins in her cupboard. She'd been a terrible hoarder, she admitted. Quentin believed it. Push came to shove, she said, she could stay in her flat for about a month and never go out, living on her tinned supplies. But fresh food would be welcome.

That was the last time he had spoken to her. Two days later, he had switched his computer on, but there was no Wi-Fi. A temporary problem, but when he tried to watch the news on the telly, that was gone too; the lights as well. Electricity was out. The switches on the fuse box did nothing to bring the power back on. The computer had been getting to the end of its battery. The water was still running, for the moment. Things would be restored in time. He was secure where he was.

These days, he locked the back door with all three locks, even when he went to the beach. In other times, he had done this only when leaving the house to return to London for some time. It made the house safe; it also condemned him to stand there longer than felt comfortable, when he wanted to get back in, fumbling with keys. On the fence, the cryptic sign, painted in white. All of the minute it took him to open the door, he had in his mind a picture of *the boys* sauntering through the garden gate, their eyes alight with mischief, their cheekbones smeared with the blood of a crucified pet, weapons over their shoulders as they came across a new fellow to have some fun with. They were out there. The thought made him fumble still more ineptly. Those may have been voices he heard, footsteps padding along the path. So far they had been illusions. Today again he was lucky. He was through the door and locking it from the inside. The house was dark and quiet. On the kitchen table there was a folded jumper where he had left it, and he put that on. He took off his flip-flops; they made a loud noise of slapping when he walked, audible from outside. He would have liked to have a coffee, but that was no longer a possibility.

Without lifting any of the blinds or opening the curtains, Quentin went barefoot through the dark bungalow. There was something new. On the mat by the front door, a cream-coloured but grubby envelope. It had been months since the post had stopped, without any explanation or justification. Now whenever anything failed, it needed no explanation. It was clear and agreed by everyone what the viral cause must be. Quentin took a pair of old blue surgical gloves from the Japanese jar on the side table and picked it up. It was crumpled and dirty; it had been carried around for some time. He took it back to his kitchen table and sat down. With a gloved finger he opened the envelope. On the surface of things it was a letter from his father. But that was unlikely. He wondered what it really was.

The people bringing this letter are coming in your direction, the letter said. They have some access to petrol, too. I don't know how. There are always going to be black-marketeers, wide boys making a good living somehow and knowing where they can get petrol. Anyway, I asked them if they could get a letter to you and at first they said no. Then a few days later, one of them comes to the old surgery and it appears that his son is in pain. Terrible pain, the wide boy says. We come to an agreement. I'll take the tooth out; he delivers this letter. That seemed fair enough to both of us. I even threw in one of the last shots of anaesthetic. I did ask if they would stop and wait until you could write a response. But the wide boy said, these days, they don't stop and wait anywhere, not for anything. Which is fair enough.

Well, son, I am in Ramsgate as ever was, except that Ramsgate is not what it was and I suppose not the rest of the world, either. I've taken a few steps and I'm

confident that I'm safe and secure here in the two upper
floors. The surgery got done over a few weeks ago but I
was expecting that. I sat it out quietly and they went
away after a bit. I've heard the carnival go by a couple of
times, a few shrieks, a few indications that things are
getting out of hand somewhere within earshot. But
nothing's come close for a while. I might be under the
protection of the wide boys now. After the last hairy
night I found a pallet of tinned beans on the floor of the
surgery, twenty-four tins. That was after I'd taken the
boy's tooth out. Payment of some kind, I suppose.
They'd ransacked the open-all-hours and burnt it, but
that was weeks ago. I can't stand baked beans, as you
may remember, even if there was some way of warming
the things up, but it was meant kindly, I suppose.

So, son, I hope you had the sense you were born with
and stayed where you were in Whitstable. I bet you're
glad of that funny little house now. If you didn't, and if
you're in London, you won't get this. But if you're there,
this is just to say that I'm here. It's not that far. I don't
know, twenty miles? I would say it was possible to walk
that if you were careful and kept an eye out for any
trouble and pop a carving knife in your knapsack, just
in case. I reckon it would make sense.

No need to let me know you're coming, I'm not
going anywhere soon.

For some time there had been a regular, timid noise from
outside. Quentin had read no sentence meant for him to read
for weeks – he shrank from remembering the last time that had
happened. The last time he had read a sentence in anyone's
handwriting meant for him had been long before that. His
father's handwriting in blue biro, on paper torn from a recep-

tionist's notepad, had absorbed him. Now he had stopped reading, his attention returned to the world; the regular tapping that had started some time ago and was continuing patiently worked its way into his awareness. After a while he understood what it was. Linda was tapping on her kitchen window, six feet from his own, trying to get his attention. He listened. The regular and patient sound continued. There was something enchanting about it, like the measured chime of a beautifully calibred instrument, a clock ticking, a pendulum swinging. He could get up and respond or he could sit and enjoy the tocking in the stillness.

The last time he had seen his father, that teller of tales, that pub raconteur, that striker-up of conversations in the park, that seducer of women, that life and, he said of himself, soul of the party whom the partygoers slid away from. The last time he had seen him. There had been a hooting in the road outside at nine on a Sunday morning. It had continued for some minutes. A neighbour had shouted, Stop that bloody row. Then his father's voice, not shouting but a raised posh drawl, posher than his usual style, I'm just attempting to rouse my fucking idle son, it said. Quentin got up. He went to the front door in his dressing-gown – it was his father, and he had chosen the smarter one of the two, the red silk paisley one.

I'll only come in, his father said, if I'm not intruding.

You're not intruding, Quentin said. Nor was he: this wasn't one of Scott's weekends.

I know what you're going to say, his father said. You're going to say, To what do I owe this pleasure.

I will if you want me to, Quentin said.

Sunday morning, you know, his father said. Out last night, I dare say. If there's a young lady in question.

I'm quite alone, Quentin said. Cup of coffee? Had breakfast?

Bad luck, his father said, coming into the house and shutting the door behind him. He wiped his feet with surgical care on the doormat. Home alone. Better luck next time. When I was your age –

I had a quiet night in, Quentin said.

– I was getting through the nurses' hostel like a knife through butter. Coffee? So long as it's not that instant muck. Those were the days, he said, sitting down. I don't suppose it would be permitted now, going up to a student nurse and saying the sort of things we used to say to get them into bed.

What sort of things did you used to say? Quentin said.

Oh, terrible things, his father said. They seemed to like it. Tell them they could do with losing ten kilos.

Yes, they know about that now, Quentin said. That pick-up technique. I don't suppose it works so well.

You don't sweat much for a fat bird, his father said. I dare say I've never had a nurse work for me who I didn't screw. They liked it, too.

They said they liked it. Then they went off to work for someone else.

True, his father said. How's that side of things, your end? I never hear you mention anyone. Ships in the night, is it? A fit bloke like you, I bet you're fighting them off. Gym bunny, isn't that the phrase? Gym bunny. I like that.

That sort of thing.

Mind you, his father said, with you it's all ornamental, isn't it. Don't suppose you've ever used those muscles to do anything but prop up a wall in a bar. When was the last time you lifted a spade? Never, I bet.

Where did my old dad ever hear the expression 'gym bunny'? Quentin said.

There's things to be said for girlfriends, his father said. And wives. Maybe you want to ask one of them back. A regular thing.

I'll let you know, Quentin said. Here's your coffee. What do I owe this honour to?

His father gave him a faintly startled look. In turn, he had got the phrase wrong. That was not what you said. In his father's world, when you had an unexpected call, you didn't say, What do I owe this honour to, you said, To what do I owe this honour. No wonder he got a startled look. In a moment his father answered, but uncertainly, from a distance. Perhaps that was what the whole thing was like, watching his father and then trying to do it, but getting it slightly wrong. His father's confident phrase was garbled; his father's loud checked trousers emerged as chinos in beige; his father's confident independence was a solitary existence. Most of all there were those ways with nurses, and his father's readiness to discuss his triumphs. If anything occupied the same place in Quentin's life, they were approached in city-centre bars, silver, mirrored and sumptuous with imperial purple. Sometimes Quentin would come up with the words, I don't suppose you would. The strange thing was that these people quite often would. Quentin knew that the expression 'I don't suppose you would' did not give off the aura of sexual power, said to be indispensable when approaching these people. Sometimes he had approached people virtually, over a phone app, and there he knew he was more confident. You could curate yourself, control what you allowed yourself to say, edit what you looked like (biceps, pecs), summarize yourself with bleak and dishonest efficiency. It did not seem to make much difference, whether this edited Quentin approached these people, or the real one went up to them in public and began by saying, I don't suppose you would. Perhaps this was the one clear connection between his father and him: when he went up to one of these people, though he spoke in a diffident style, still these people often gave in and smiled, accepted an invitation as readily as his father's nurses. Shy, aren't you, they quite often said. Big lad like you, too. The difference was that when Quentin was naked in front of another naked stranger in a locked room, he knew and was assured of his power. He did not believe his father knew the same of himself.

These people. Even talking about it to himself Quentin did not want to use the more exact description, these men.

It was none of anyone's business who he went to bed with. It was a private matter. Of course you could not say that. It was tantamount to admitting you were a homosexual. So he never spoke of it, and his father was probably the only person who could have asked a direct question about it. His father could be answered directly, because soon he would lose interest. He would turn to his favourite subject: himself. Quentin could emulate him, but in the end he would be a peculiar shadow of an imitation, in which something, who could say what, was amiss. What do I owe this pleasure to, His father would look at him. He could see something was not quite right, but he had no real way of describing the evidence he had. What would that evidence have been? One of those men. Scott, perhaps. They had been working up to that moment of explanation, of the unveiling of the self-evident. But in general these men were not the material out of which husbands were made. They appeared in Quentin's life, and then after a few hours, they went away without wanting to do it again. In any case they had gone away for good now. There were no apps, since there was no way of charging your smartphone, and even if you could have charged it, there was no network service. There were no bars to meet people: no catching of the eye, no way of turning aside shyly or of walking over and offering to buy a drink, no drink to offer to buy. No one would come within twelve feet of another man, these days. He had no idea where Scott was, with the scattering of freckles across his broad shoulders, the lecher-

ous innocent smile in his broad ginger's face. Sex with a
stranger, if you followed the instructions of the government,
would look like two midshipmen flailing, practising semaphore
from either end of a poop deck. The last instructions of the
government. Nobody knew what they were now instructing.

That Sunday morning had turned out to have a purpose, one
quite familiar to Quentin. His father had sat at the kitchen
table, and his conversation had gone from the nurses he had
known to the garden that one of those nurses had had. His
belief had always been that women who cared for cooking were
putting themselves to too much trouble to please a man; those
who cared for gardening were planning to hide themselves
away. The cooking ones would cry when you left them, and the
gardening ones wouldn't notice you'd gone. There was a fat
nurse called Iris; Jamaican; liked tree ferns. The things he could
tell Quentin about Iris. And then the conversation went its way.
His father was planning to go to a garden centre that morning.

Of course if you don't want to come, but if you didn't have
anything better to do, his father said.

I don't mind, Quentin said. Use my ornamental muscles to
lift a plant pot.

I tell you what, his father said. I don't have any cash on me.
Can you lend me two hundred quid, say three hundred?

I don't have that, Quentin said. I don't suppose I ever have
more than fifty quid in my wallet.

Doesn't matter, Quentin's father said. We could stop at a
cashpoint on our way to the garden centre.

Yes, we could, Quentin said shortly. We'll stop at a cashpoint so you can get out some money.

Quentin's father stared; scratched the back of his head;
richly gurgled at this absurdity. Come on, Quent, he said.
Come on. Come off it. It's just a loan. Won't hurt you. What's
it to you? A mere three hundred.

Quentin took his father's mug from him and placed it, with a great deal of precision, in the sink. He could feel the tightness of his lips. He believed that his father now owed him something like two thousand pounds. Sometimes it had been a spur-of-the-moment thing, the request for the loan, sometimes a hangdog bit of begging, his father's eyes mournful, sometimes jauntily open about being in a bit of a pickle. Quentin didn't think he was the one his father went to first, either. Not his first port of call, as he would have said. God knows how much he owed those nurses, his old mistresses.

Let's go, Quentin said.

We'll go in your car, his father said, as Quentin locked his front door.

This is an awful car, he said, buckling up. I can't imagine what possessed you.

Honestly, I'm ashamed that a son of mine should drive something so dreary, he said. The car was drumming along the A road. This sort of beige cockroach. Doodling along interminably. I just cannot imagine going into a showroom and saying, That's the very car for me.

Well, it's a good job it's my car and not yours, then, Quentin said. I can't understand how you never have any money.

Oh, we're there, are we? Quentin's father said.

I don't really want to know, Quentin said.

Obligations, Quentin's father said. Long-standing commitments. Necessary expenditure. It all builds up.

Alimony and child support, Quentin said.

Don't be absurd, his father said. Here's one, this petrol station.

Quentin stopped; went over; returned.

Out of action, he said.

Turned you down, did it? his father said. Must be awful when that happens. Did you try a different card? Not many people know this, but you can get cash on a credit card from one of those machines.

My account is fine, Quentin said. The machine wasn't functioning. There's another one on the way.

Way where?

The garden centre, Quentin said. You wanted to go to the garden centre.

Oh, yes, the garden centre. Forget my own name next, his father said. Yes, the garden centre. Thought I'd put some bulbs in. A shrub or two. Forsythia. Someone was telling me about forsythia.

I've heard of that, Quentin said.

On the other hand, his father said, we're a bit later than I'd like. Let's take a look at the situation when we get there. Garden centre on a Sunday morning, it's the middle classes' preferred outing.

And ours, of course.

Not mine, his father said. I tell you what. Once we've got the wonga, we take a butcher's at the state of things. Massive queue and we won't bother. These rules, they're so absurd. Only twenty customers allowed at any one time. Keep forty metres away from the nearest human. Wear a mask and another mask on top of that – that was what they were saying on the telly yesterday. Never heard anything so absurd. Result: enormous queue outside garden centre, middle classes full of rage. No thanks, buster.

Let's see, Quentin said. Look on the bright side. They might all have decided to stay at home. Or they might all have died.

That would be a bright side, his father said. I don't know what you think. This fifth wave, so-called. Killing everybody. I don't believe it. Do you know anyone who's died from it? You had it, two years ago. Did you die? It's all nonsense.

Probably nonsense, Quentin said. It was always quicker to agree with his father, and give him some money halfway through the conversation. Here we go.

They turned into the car park of the big Sainsbury's. There were certainly cashpoints there. The supermarket would not open for another hour, but it was surprising to see how few cars there were in the car park, scattered around the marked-up tarmac expanse, like the last few balls in a game of snooker.

Park in the disabled, his father said. It's closest.

I'll do that, Quentin said.

Surely the lights should be on in the supermarket by now. He parked the car by the cashpoint machines and got out. There was nobody inside the building that he could see, and everything was dark. He went to the cashpoint machines and put his card in. He followed the familiar sequence, but the machine was unable to fulfil his request. He tried the other machine, but that had no money, either; after the third had failed him, he tried another request, asking what the balance in his current account was. The machine was unable to carry out his request. He returned to the car.

Nothing's working, he said. Bad luck.

What do you mean, his father said.

Quentin explained.

You're doing something wrong, his father said. Give me your PIN and I'll try.

Quentin ignored this. He started the car and reversed out of the space.

Do you still want to go to the garden centre, he said.

Yes, of course, his father said. Why wouldn't I.

They chose a face-saving dahlia. There was no queue; there were no customers. The owner was the only person working at the garden centre, and she stood well back, telling them to leave ten pounds by the till. Quentin was about to do so.

Just take it, his father said. Ten quid. Absurd.

Ten pounds, the owner said. She was a woman with a grey tight crop; an expression of great uncertainty crossed her eyes.

Taking advantage, his father said. You'll need that ten pounds. Let's go.

It was with a sensation of behaving, for once, like his father, that Quentin walked after him, still holding the face-saving dahlia.

I'm calling the police, the owner shouted after them, bravely but without convincing anyone. I'm calling the police. I'm calling them now.

Tell that bitch to shut up, Quentin's father said. At the door to the car park Quentin handed the dahlia to his father. He turned with a sense of light-hearted possibility, and went back to the bleating woman at the till. He reached out and, quite hard, slapped the woman's face. He couldn't remember the last time he'd slapped anyone; perhaps he never had. The woman took her face in her own hands. He turned and went back to his father, whose eyes were gleaming.

That's the ticket, his father said. Silly bitch.

He handed the plant back to Quentin. They left, and heard the door of the business being locked behind them. They drove back to Quentin's house, not talking much, but with a light-heartedness in the car as they pointed out new things to each other. All that work in the gym; all that iron and weight; and now he had hit someone with his useful muscles. Around them, the quiet of a Kent Sunday morning had become the quiet of something new.

Not got any petrol in a can, have you? Quentin's father said. They got out of Quentin's car. A bit short.

Doesn't matter, he said after Quentin had apologized. There's probably enough in the tank to get me back at least.

I'm sure there is. Better set off. Good to see you. Don't punch anyone I wouldn't punch.

That was the last time Quentin had seen his father, though he knew he had got back. One of his father's usual reassuring phone calls, full of blame, that he was quite safe and secure, had come that evening. There was a can of petrol he'd forgotten about in the corner of the garage, apparently. So that was all hunky-dory. Quentin wasn't sure he believed in the can of petrol. But there was no way of buying any more, or of getting any cash from the machines. The systems had gone down and had stayed down. It was that day, or maybe the Monday, that he'd seen a supermarket with its window smashed; that Friday when he wondered why nobody was doing anything about it. He left the face-saving dahlia in its nursery pot outside the back door, not watering or planting it. In a few days it had died. The police never came to arrest him for assault.

He was still thinking about the letter his father had somehow got to him. There was a figure in his garden, not moving, tapping shyly at the window. He gave a small spasm of alarm.

It's me, a voice said. It was not a thug or the scout of a gang; it was not a creature from fiction or fantasy, though the faces of the undead were no longer impossible. It was only Linda, who lived next door. One day it would be the scout of a gang.

Hey, Quentin said. You made me jump. He opened the french windows, staying in the sitting room.

You had a visitor, Linda said. Or visitors.

It was just someone posting a letter, Quentin said.

Unusual, Linda said. Unusual these days, anyway. We wondered, me and … me and Simon.

Whenever Linda said her son's name, she paused and collected herself, looked away. Quentin wondered what Simon's name had originally been, before he had decided to change it to that of someone thirty years older, one so redolent of malt loaf for tea and Ladybird books about the lives of famous scientists. There was no need to be rude to Linda. She had a fair amount to put up with, as everyone did, of course.

I don't know who they were, Quentin said. They were just delivering a message from my dad. He's in Ramsgate, apparently.

That's not far, Linda said. That's where my other son lives.

I'm thinking of walking there, Quentin said. He was thinking of Scott in his little fisherman's cottage, painted pale green. He might be there, if he wasn't in Kentish Town. He might have holed up like anyone else might.

Walking to Ramsgate, Linda said. I suppose it's possible. See your dad. Makes sense.

He wants me to, Quentin said.

Ah, that's sweet, Linda said. I wonder how Luke's doing. I hope he's all right.

There was something performed and suggestive about those last sentences, like a cue in a play. They sounded unnatural in Linda, who had never been known to direct much affectionate speculation towards her elder son; that one had, Quentin believed, run a small drug-dealing business in Ramsgate, using ten-year-olds to deliver envelopes of cocaine to his WhatsApp customers. He had given 'a number' to Quentin a couple of years ago, and Quentin had given it to Scott, who had used it occasionally. Luke had made out it was the number of a friend, but the matt black BMW he drove had had to come from some source. WhatsApp had gone the way of everything else, into the long night of a small black screen, and the sources of drugs must have long run dry, and nobody had any cash to hand over, and the ten-year-olds on their bikes had found other things to do, other masters to work for. Or Luke had found other things to occupy them in his service. Luke was probably all right; he would always be all right. Linda had never wondered about him before, and now she said she hoped he was all right, over in Ramsgate, to see what Quentin would offer to do.

Linda, I can't go round Ramsgate trying to find Luke, Quentin said. It was best to be frank.

I wasn't asking, thank you, Linda said.

It sounds a complete shitshow, Quentin said. Worse than here. If I go –

Oh, you ought to go, Linda said. You've only got one dad.

– if I go, I'll go straight to him, Quentin said. Then take it from there.

This was not quite honest: Quentin would go to Scott's house first. If he went.

I wouldn't ask you to do anything I wouldn't do, Linda said. Her dress was clean, but faded and not ironed, and loose-hanging. She was still plump, but had been fat; she had lost weight and had gone deep into her clothes cupboard to find this floral pinafore. She looked at him, guilelessly.

I'm sure he's fine, Quentin said, not caring. You shouldn't worry. He can look after himself.

What if, Linda said, when you went you took – you took Simon. I wouldn't want to ask Simon to go on his own. But two of you, that's different. Once you get to Ramsgate you can go to your dad's and he goes to Luke's place.

It's a long walk, Quentin said.

It's nothing to a boy that age, Linda said. It's safer for you too. They're not going to go for two big lads in the way they would for somebody on their own.

I don't think so, Quentin said.

Please, Linda said. I'd give him some digestive sandwiches to eat on the way. The digestive biscuits are holding up still and there's still a bit of cheese to pop between them. You wouldn't have to give him any food on the way.

Linda.

The fact is, Linda said, the fact is, he's doing my head in. All day long! All that … She made a duckbill with her right hand; made it open and shut repeatedly, the old gesture for incessant gabble. A generation older, and she'd have said rabbit-rabbit-rabbit.

Well, I can see that, Quentin said. You're not tempting me to take him.

But in the end it was agreed. Perhaps it was for the sake of Scott. For hours he would be walking in the direction where Scott might be, but there were other possibilities to mull over. In those hours, if he were alone, those possibilities would be mulled over and over. What might have happened to Scott.

He didn't remember having this degree of investment when Scott was there. They had met in London. Scott was three hundred metres away from Quentin's place in Kentish Town – an estimation by the app, one Sunday afternoon, which turned out to be more or less correct.

what are you into
the usual stuff
you look hot. want to see you in those Speedos
that was in Sardinia last month
still got the suntan
ha ha just the freckles
got a thing for a ginger
oh it's like that is it
yeah
okay come round and objectify me
address
just getting to that

And afterwards – lying there after Quentin had taken a shower and Scott was still freckled and sweaty and smelling good, his white sheets rumpled, the palm of his hand rough on Quentin's chest, his fingers idly tweaking Quentin's nipples, one after the other.

I've never fucked a Quentin before, Scott said.

Was it a wonderful new experience for you?

When I was at school, Scott said, Quentin was what you said instead of bender. Oi, you big Quentin.

That's weird, Quentin said. What we said in the playground was Oi, you big Scott, but that was only if you wanted to be punched in the face.

So what did you call a big Scot from Scotland?

We said, Oi, Jock. I like your balls.

Yeah, my big ginger balls. I stopped shaving them.

I noticed. Big ginger caveman appeal.

Quentin got up, making a regretful noise, spreading his hands as if in apology. He went to the little sofa at the end of the bed, and picked up the pair of jeans. They must have been in a hurry for him to drop his jeans like that, but there was nothing as unsexy as watching your date fold his clothes as he stripped. He pulled the jeans on, but something was wrong. Scott was watching him, laughter bright in his blue eyes.

Do you always go commando, he said.

Sometimes, Quentin said.

Yeah, but do you always go commando in other people's 501s.

Oh, fuck. Sorry.

You looked like you were having some difficulty. What size are you? I'm twenty-eight.

Thirty.

Lardarse.

Fuck off, Quentin said, but cheerfully. He dropped Scott's jeans on the floor, and put his own on. He carefully tucked his cock and balls in, feeling a little revival of energy, of blood. Scott's trainers were there, too, a pair of silver Onitsuka Tigers, and just to make a kind of joke, Quentin started to put them on.

Oi, Scott said. Get your trotters out of me prized disco slippers.

Same size this time, Quentin said. They fit me.

I'm not sharing my shoes with anyone, Scott said. Athlete's foot.

Verrucas, Quentin said. This was good.

You're a good fuck.

Thanks. You too.

What are you doing tonight?

No plans. Well, yes. I've got this house on the coast. Bit of a new thing. I thought I'd get in the car and drive out there for the weekend.

Whereabouts?

So that was how they established where they lived. Scott's flat in London was three hundred metres from Quentin's; it was a mess, every time Quentin went round there, and in the end Quentin said, Look, just come round here. I can't stand picking stuff up and having to clean the kitchen before I can make a cup of tea.

In Kent, they lived twenty miles from each other, Quentin in Whitstable and Scott in Ramsgate. He'd been once to Scott's – a little fisherman's cottage with unwashed dishes a week old in the sink. I could have got something a bit bigger, Scott said, but I liked this one. Usually Scott came over to Quentin's. He'd come over eight, maybe ten times, coming on a Saturday night, going back on Sunday, about lunchtime. Nobody knew about him. If he left the house late enough in the morning, nobody would think he'd spent the night. It was the first time Quentin had had somebody regular, leaving his stuff in the expectation he'd be back. At some point he supposed he'd have either to tell Scott he was a secret, or tell everyone else about Scott. He was at this point when everything changed. Scott was supposed to come over one Saturday night, but he hadn't. He could have been in London, or he could have been in Ramsgate. A pair of jeans and a couple of T-shirts belonging to Scott were in the wardrobe, a bottle of the shampoo Scott couldn't live without in the bathroom cupboard. Had he been – was he his boyfriend? Was that what he had been about to ask, the last time they'd seen each other? Boyfriend, he sang internally, scornful in his tone. What a word. All his feelings for Scott were from the time after he had gone from his life, along with everyone else who lived more than a mile distant.

It was those feelings, he supposed, that made him give way to Linda. The boy should be there, ready to leave, at six the next morning. She agreed; and the next morning, there he was.

From where he stood he could smell Simon. The boy had prepared himself for company, or perhaps that was what he always did, poured deodorant over himself. He would get to the end of his stocks soon at this rate. Quentin never used deodorant: he thought the metallic smell given off by paranoid devotion much worse than a body an hour after swimming in the sea. Simon was looking in another direction and yet somehow assessing Quentin closely. He began to talk. Simon was a boy who liked to have his conversation prepared in advance. There was no point in saying anything in response. Nothing would knock him from his prepared speech, protecting him against the unscripted contribution. In a few minutes – Quentin knew this from experience – he would come to the end of what he had prepared, and they would be able to talk in an ordinary way. For the moment he talked, and what he said, he had thought over in his bedroom. Quentin locked the house. They left the little garden, and Quentin locked the garden gate. They started to walk towards the sea. Quentin looked about, hardly listening, for any sign of strangers, any sign of trouble.

This is very good of you, Simon said.

No trouble, Quentin said. We'll be company for each other.

It really is so strange, Simon said. When one thinks how remote our lives before have become. I wonder whether they shall ever return. Do you know the thing that brought it home to me? I remembered the last time I saw an actor on a stage, a live actor on a stage. Do you remember the last time you were in a theatre? I certainly do.

Quentin did not remember the last time he was in a theatre, the lights lowering, sitting close to a human being he knew nothing of, watching a paid actor, a flesh-coloured blemish of a microphone hovering above his face, advance to the foot-lights as the music swelled. It had been a treat that had been inflicted on him. He said nothing.

I love the theatre, Simon went on. Perhaps it would be better to say I loved the theatre.

He paused.

Perhaps it would, Quentin said lightly. The boy was coming too close to him, less than the ten feet required. Simon looked at him as if a member of a congregation had made a response from the pews to a point made in a sermon.

I loved the theatre, Simon said. But that's all over now. The last time I went it was with Mummie, for my birthday. I had seen it announced, a new production of *Uncle Vanya*, you know, the play by Chekhov. I had never seen it. I wonder now – did something within me say to me, Go, go, go. Go to see *Uncle Vanya*, this time, this production, because if you pass up this chance, you will never see *Uncle Vanya*, not as long as you live. I wonder: will that be the last ever production of that …

Simon trailed away. Perhaps he had been about to say, That great play by the Russian master, but had felt, on bringing out the first half of the sentence, that he would be defeated by it. In any case he let his sentence trail away.

Did you enjoy it, Quentin said.

I saw that it was about to be staged, Simon said, his confidence returning. And I begged, begged Mummie to take me to see it as a birthday treat. I thought so carefully about everything, the whole outing. It had to be a matinee performance, of course, because of the trains back home. Mummie wanted to take me out for lunch in London before, but I thought we would have to rush, and I prevailed on her to go for an early supper instead, and we would discuss the play. You can imagine that wasn't very successful! However, I planned what I should wear, and made it clear in my mind what train we should take, and what the best route to the theatre would be – I was determined that we should not be late. In fact we should in the event be almost an hour early. We had been to London before, many times, naturally, so we took shelter in a Pret a Manger a street away from the theatre. Pret a Manger – how ordinary those sandwiches seemed, just two years ago! I remember every detail of that day, now. I remember I had a bacon, lettuce and tomato sandwich. Mummie had something with avocado in it. We both had a sparkling water, too. We decided to eat no more than a sandwich there before the theatre because we would have a proper supper later on. It is one of Mummie's rules – it was one of Mummie's rules – that one should never eat in a restaurant, a proper restaurant I mean, twice in one day. That was the day I discovered this rule of Mummie's. The question had never arisen before.

Silence fell. They were walking by now at the top of the grass slope that fell towards the stony beach, divided by groynes, and the almost unmoving sea. There was nobody around, as far as Quentin could see, at most some kind of dark movement half a mile off, at the water's edge, and that could be anything. Simon had lost his thread, his prepared spiel.

So you went to see the play, Quentin said.

Yes, Simon said gratefully. The single thing I remember from that performance was this. I know it may seem inexplicable, extraordinary, bizarre to recall only one thing, and that so unimportant a thing. The star of the show – the *vedette* if I am using the word correctly, the draw, the big name in lights, the Vanya, you would have seen him many times in television series and in films – was utterly magnetic on stage, in person. At one point the niece says something to him, asking him what he feels his life should consist of, what steps he hopes to take towards a marvellous and fulfilled future. And the star started to raise his hands as if in despair, but the gesture was altogether too much for him, or for his character; the character lifted his arms a little from his sides, then let them drop again. Like a penguin, you might say. It was very like a penguin. I remember – I gasped. I gulped with laughter. It was the thought of a penguin. A penguin playing Chekhov's ruined hero with no future. Mummie looked at me strangely, disapprovingly. But that is what I remember, on that day when, we all failed to understand, there was no future; the gesture that Uncle Vanya made, so noncommittal and such a failed gesture, when he is asked about his own future.

Just for a second Quentin thought there was no more to say. Simon had stopped speaking, and also stopped walking. Quentin had gone a few steps further before he noticed, and turned to see Simon gazing out to sea. It was a bright day, hazy at the horizon, and the wind turbines were lost to sight. Their positions were awkward. It appeared that Simon was oblivious to Quentin; his long gaze, his faint sway forwards and backwards, signified *lost in thought* as it might have been taught in an A-level drama course. Quentin stayed where he was, and after an interval Simon performed awareness, a brittle sort of smile, a shrug. They started walking again, and Simon returned to his theme.

It was so wonderful, he said. Even if it had been followed by another trip to the theatre, the next week, and another, and another, it would have been wonderful. And worth it for that gesture of Vanya alone. But now, recognizing that that experience may be the last ever such experience, it makes it so ... so ... so ... sometimes heartbreaking is the only word. To know that there is no future, for us or for Vanya. So uncommitted. Such a failed gesture. Heartbreaking.

Quentin felt he had not been sent the necessary script for this particular scene and, in any case, had been thrown into something that would have required a more capable performer. He did his best.

Didn't you want to be an actor yourself? he said. Your mum told me, some time.

I only wish, Simon said. I mean, yes, I did.

Hard to succeed in that profession, Quentin said. Or so they say.

I'd have liked to have a go, Simon said. I did A-level drama. I was Willy Loman in an excerpt, I did him in my underpants, showing his vulnerability. I got a B.

Well, Quentin said.

There seemed nothing more for either of them to say. Simon gave the impression of having been stuck with an inadequate feed who had never learnt his lines. Solitary, he had constructed this scene or something like it in detail; perhaps an argument where he came out victorious, his virtue and his talent indisputably recognized. But he could not do it all on his own, and Quentin could see that he had not imagined who he would be arguing with, who he would triumph over. When it came to the point, it was only Quentin from next door, who was not much of an adversary. You could not strike postures quite on your own.

The true and beautiful tomorrow, Simon said. His voice was different – hushed, growling, portentous. He must be quoting from the part he'd had. All that is gonna be taken away from us. Where shall we go? How shall we live? We must go on. We shall go on. I loved doing that bit. I don't know why. I could just imagine when it got to the point of having an audience in that, I mean, how could they not burst into tears?

Did you get an audience in, Quentin said.

Well, it was just friends and family, two each, Simon said. And not the whole play, so it was a bit disappointing. Mummie is so hopeless. She promised she'd bring her friend Doreen, then forgot to ask her, so that was a seat lost. Lost for ever.

He raised the back of his hand to his forehead in a practised, ironic performing pose.

And then, of course, I said afterwards, What did you think, and she just said, Very nice, Simon. And that was it. Hopeless. Anyway.

Quentin's sense of the geography of his setting had hardened and clarified in the last weeks. So much might depend on it. The orange-brick development he lived in, the sixty or so bungalows, had been built on a patch of land in the 1930s. Its borders were clear, and tightly defined. Beyond them in one direction bigger, square Victorian houses dotted with what he supposed were historic survivors, like the house titled The Old Forge behind a hedge of untended, leggy, scraggily yellow-leaved rose bushes. In the other direction it opened up, a stretch of bright grass the width of a cricket pitch between a line of uncared-for hotels and the slope down to the shingle beach. The line of hotels bore incomplete names, a dented signboard suggesting vacancies, windows that had needed a coat of paint before and needed one now. In some a large arrangement of dried flowers gave off an aura of dust, even at two hundred yards. They were out of the estate they lived on, and on the path along the green, now shaggy and uncared-for.

There was a sense of a border being crossed, and with some apparent inevitability two figures ambled forward, a hundred yards ahead, to intervene in their path. They had the look of bored, confident officials; perhaps that was now what they were. They were both women, efficiently dressed in black; one wore what might have been a biker's jacket, hanging open loosely, like a pair of doors on broken hinges. One was white; the other, the one in the biker jacket, mixed race, her hair cropped close and bleached blonde. They watched Quentin and Simon approach, patiently, taking charge of the situation.

Hi there, Quentin said.

On a walk, are we, the white woman said. She had a low, harmonious voice of some authority, a manager or a senior teacher in real life.

How far are you going, the other said.

It's a nice day, Simon said uncertainly.

Where have you come from, the bleached-blonde one said. She stood with her legs apart, her arms folded across her chest.

About half a mile in that direction, Quentin said. We live there.

Live on the Sunward estate, do we? the white woman said, almost jeering. Quentin had heard it called that; he wondered where the name came from. What's your road, the one you live on?

What is this?

The biker woman took a step forward, into the safe zone around Quentin and Simon.

You know what's happening, she said. We're having to look after ourselves. Keep an eye on who's turning up. Anyone could say they live where you say you do.

Annabella Avenue, Simon said impatiently. Where do you live, then?

We live over there, the white woman said. I live in one house and she lives in another. A word of advice. If you need a walk in future, stay somewhere you actually live, walk round that bit. People are a bit – what's the expression – a bit on edge. Trigger happy. If I were you I'd get a bit of air and then go back wherever you've come from. All right then. On your way.

Yeah, off you pop, Simon said. You two – off you pop. No hurry. No reply came, and they walked away with a sense of being found unworthy of the rejoinder. I know them, Simon said. I mean I don't know them but I know the type. They love a rule, they'll make something up. There was a kid at school who was always saying – this is at infant school I'm talking about – there was a sort of bit round the back where no one could see you, and this kid, his name was Ryan, he just said one day, This bit's only for year four and then only if we say you can.

What did people do?

That was the strange thing. They mostly just accepted it, like it was a new rule. Then it was about a month later one of the teachers got wind of it and she got hold of Ryan Crawford and made him apologize to the whole school in Assembly. But I don't think anyone went round to the bit that was only for year fours anyway, or maybe just the once, out of bravado. Why was I saying this?

People in authority.

Oh, yeah. Most people wouldn't have said, Off you pop, to those women, they'd have just done something meek, apologized and called them Officer.

I rather admired how well you lied. Annabella Avenue. Not telling them the right road.

I'm like that. I never wanted to do anything just because

someone told me to do it. Or tell the truth to someone just because they've got a uniform on.

If everyone was like that.

The world would be a better place, I know, Simon said, in some excitement.

If everyone was like that, I was going to say, Quentin said, then we'd be in trouble. You have to have rules that people agree to obey or everyone would take to shitting on the beach and not caring.

Nobody's going to do that.

They've already started doing that.

How do you mean?

It was a warm day by now. It would once have been described as a beautiful day for a walk, looking out to sea at the wind turbines. They glittered in the sun; the clarity startled the eyes and made them ache. Privation had got him used to inconvenience; it was only now that Quentin remembered he had packed an old pair of sunglasses, that the sunglasses still worked perfectly. One day he would drop them, or step on them, and there would be no means of repairing or replacing them, but that day had not happened yet. Without stopping walking, he reached behind him, tugged open the side pocket of his rucksack, pulled out his sunglasses and put them on. Simon watched him all this while as if preparing for a role. He started to tell the story.

So this morning. I like to go for a swim, Quentin said. In the sea. It's nice. It's one of the things that made me buy a house down here.

I wondered about that, Simon said. Me and Mummie. We wondered why someone like you would want to buy a house down here in Whitstable.

I don't see why not. Someone like you. What – no, forget it. I'm someone who likes a bit of fresh air in the morning. Every day I go out for a swim, unless it's really cold, and sometimes I still do even in January, it won't kill you. There's hardly ever anyone around, towel and flip-flops on the groynes, straight in, bish bosh, five hundred yards out to sea, back again, straight out, and that's me set up for the day. Lovely. Today, though. I'm going down to the sea and there's this old man standing at the top of the beach, looking around, nervous. And when he sees that I'm going down to the sea just about there, he says, Go away, very cross, trying to impress me. And I'm about to say, No, you go away, it's not your bit of beach, but then I see that his old wife it must be is down there, right by the sea's edge. You know what she's doing? Having a shit on the beach. Her skirt's hoicked up and she's crouching down and she's having a shit.

How disgusting, Simon said.

Yeah, Quentin said. Perhaps the story had finished. It lacked something.

I can't stand swimming, Simon said. I couldn't go in the sea because of that. You're going to come up with your nose against someone's turd. I couldn't bear it in the swimming pool they used to take us to because of the chlorine. They used to put loads of chlorine in to kill all the cockroaches. It was someone's job to go round with a net in the morning scooping out all the cockroaches that had fallen in and drowned in the night.

Maybe not, Quentin said, thinking that he'd heard this about many different swimming pools.

Someone who worked there told me. And the business with the towels in the changing room after.

What business?

The flicking business, Simon said. They get your towel wet and then they flick it at you, hard. It really hurt. Maybe you would have been one of the ones doing the flicking.

Someone like me, Quentin said.

Yeah, maybe, someone like you. Wait, what do you mean?

That's twice you've said that – I'm one of those people, people different from you. First it was someone who shouldn't be living in Whitstable, then it was towel flicking. I don't know why you're so keen to think I'm in some kind of different box from you.

Simon paused in his walk; he fiddled with the left strap on his rucksack for a full minute. He would not engage Quentin's gaze, hidden behind his sunglasses. Quentin waited; not like someone waiting patiently, but like someone performing the possibility of patience, his arms folded like a schoolteacher's and his dark-glazed inspection level and unfaltering.

That's better, Simon said. It was driving me mad. What were you saying? Oh, well, yes, but you are, aren't you? In a sort of different box from people like us?

People like you. Just you, I mean.

Well, I won't go into it, Simon said.

What Quentin said next was exactly the right thing. He had sometimes seen the statement from far off, heard of it being made by others and had even listened to it. But in his recollection he had never said what now came to him as exactly the right thing; he had never told another person, man or woman, that he was homosexual. Of course it had been comfortably and lucidly established that this was the case on many occasions, established by the immediate circumstance, in bedrooms, in cyberspace, in the showers of the Kentish Town gym at a quiet time in the morning, but the moments when it might have been necessary to tell people relied on a renunciation of purpose, and Quentin had always believed that disinterest and ignorance might have a necessary connection, that, in short, if someone didn't need to know, they wouldn't be told. Most people did not need to know, and most people were not told. But now here was someone of perfect disinterest

– Simon was pudgy and nervous-looking, his hair an ugly home-dyed blond, his voice fluting, his feet miniature, his shoulders narrow, his hands fluttering and his teeth crooked. He would never be in those immediate circumstances where no explanation needed to be made, and before, he would not be told. Now, however, everything had changed. It didn't matter, today, what he said to this boy, his next-door neighbour. He might as well. He said it.

The thing is, I'm gay, Quentin said. Like you. So there you go.

Simon gratifyingly gawped. You're gay? You never are.

Quentin modestly inclined his head. The reactions of another were things he had not experienced. Once, in one of those speechless revelations, there had been a reaction, as he unrolled his Speedos down his thighs, like a knot of pastry across a hard board, stood upright in the showers of the swimming pool to explain to the other man in it, a muscular Black man with chest muscles rounded, tight and glossy as the lungs within, what he was and what he wanted. The man had sunk to his knees, but before he did so, he said one of two surprising things – Quentin could not now recall. He had said either, Oh, I knew it, or Oh, I'd never have thought you were – but whichever it was, and it was the surprise in his own reaction that Quentin remembered most clearly, he had said, Why? The man had said one last thing before they began, and again, though now Quentin remembered the words perfectly, their significance was beyond discovery. The man had said, That butterfly stroke of yours, with what was surely amusement, and had sunk without further explanation to take Quentin's erection in his hoop-round mouth. That butterfly stroke of his: it was what Quentin was proud of, the butterfly stroke, churning up the pool, like a dying salmon, the stroke of pure manly egotism, not caring about lanes or territories or others' right of space in the water, not venturing beyond its own display, a display, it might be thought, a mating display. The man's name was never learnt, and afterwards, once he had rinsed his mouth direct from the shower, spat out the residue of spunk and water cheerfully at Quentin's feet – itself a display of sheer manly competence that might have encouraged Quentin into a repeat – he had just raised his hand, said, See you, mate, and taken himself off into that other world of dryness, clothing, properties, and disguise, his red Speedos for the moment like a rag in his big hand, his purple erection waving with erratic bravado before him as if signalling in the direction of the next one. What he had meant by That butterfly stroke of yours would never be explained; perhaps that nobody could perform manliness to such a degree without it being nothing but that, a performance that no straight man could be bothered with. Or perhaps it was innocent. The expression of one good swimmer's admiration for another, just before he remembered he was supposed to fellate him.

Simon's response was not familiar to him, but any response would not have been familiar. Quentin mildly spread his hands.

How can you be …

Well, I am, Quentin said.

Mummie thought you were getting over some girlfriend, Simon said. Or a divorce you didn't want to talk about. She's quite curious. We've talked you over. But you're not.

I don't really see how I can convince you if you won't take my word, Quentin said. The boy had been inspecting him, but now he looked away again, out to sea. What Quentin said had touched some nerve, and of course he understood exactly how the boy might have wanted him to convince him by demonstration, out there on the empty sward of grass above the beach, in the sunlight, like lambs.

You're not, Simon said again. Your clothes don't fit. No gay man would buy a pair of jeans that didn't fit him. Look at yours. They're too short! No, I know where you're coming from. There was this thing in school the last year I was there, people saying they were bisexual or if they couldn't manage that, they were queer. Capital Q Queer. All these boys had spent the last five years making my life a perfect misery and now they were capital Q Queer. Of course they didn't actually do anything, that would be too much, be reasonable, you big poof, but they said they were still defining their sexuality and it was cool to be Queer. Their girlfriends loved it. Once Max Edwards kissed Winston Yip in the common room for a dare, with tongues. That was as far as it ever went. So, yeah. You mean like that, you're open to the experience of being seen as cool.

You know, Quentin said, that time might have gone. Saying you were things that you aren't for the effect of it. I might as well say what I am and, I promise you, I'm what I say I am. These jeans fit fine.

Yeah, Simon said. Maybe that's right. They're going to come for people like me, too. Now everything's finished and there's nothing but people taking care of themselves, standing in the street with an iron bar waiting to do what they've always wanted to. You're not going to say you're Queer or gay now. Nobody is. We're the first ones they're going to come for when they're bored.

I don't think so, Quentin said. We're not at that point yet.

We soon will be, Simon said. Max Edwards and Winston Yip aren't telling people they're Queer any more. They've got a choice and they've got more sense than that. I don't have a choice. It doesn't matter whether I've got more sense than that.

I don't ... Quentin said, but his sentence somehow faltered, and the image of Scott came to his mind; not Scott's face at first, but most immediately, his broad freckled shoulders giving a flex, the pepper-sprinkle of the back of his neck, the shaved back of his ginger skull. His impertinent little ears. Then in Quentin's mind he turned, and half a lazy blue-eyed face smiled.

That's why I'm going to Ramsgate, he said. See how my boyfriend's doing.

I thought you were going to see your dad, Simon said.

I might look in on the Dentist, Quentin said. But mostly it's the boyfriend.

How awfully interesting, Simon said, returning a little to his old rehearsed manner. He didn't want to hear about any boyfriend.

Ahead of them, a hundred yards away on the path above the beach and sea, there was a small human figure. The sun was shining directly at them, and only the strange proportions could at first be seen, squashed and big-headed. The figure turned and started to walk with an odd drunken totter. The size of it became clear. It was a very small child, no more than three years old. They came up to it, and it looked at them with dull, dirty attention. It was a boy, his face smeared with filth, in torn dungarees that hadn't been taken off for days. He might even have put them on himself. His bare feet were smeared with mud. He stood with one dirty fist in his mouth. He had cried quite recently.

Where's Mummie? Simon said.

The child looked, but said nothing.

Come on, Simon said. Mummie will be worrying. What's your name?

The child seemed to say Buddy, but it might have been anything.

Where do you live? Simon said. We'll take you home if you tell us where home is.

You're going to ask him his postcode in a minute, Quentin said.

Everyone knows where they live, Simon said, in a governess-like tone. It was the first thing I had drummed into me, what my address was. Come on, buddy, Mummie's worrying, she's looking for you, I bet. Have you come far? Where's Mummie?

The child looked up at Simon, then at Quentin in his sunglasses. He spoke.

Fuck Mummie, he said.

Quentin laughed. Good luck with this one, he said.

We've got to take him home, Simon said. We can't leave him here. The boys will find him and have some fun with him.

He'll be fine, Quentin said. Have some sense. If the boys find us with a toddler in tow they'll have some fun with us. We'll end up staked out on the beach or tied up and burnt at the stake. Just leave him.

I can't leave him, Simon said.

Small children are indestructible, Quentin said. If he follows us, he follows us. If not, then he probably knows where he wants to go. He stinks.

I don't know, Simon said.

Come on, Quentin said.

The small boy stayed where he was for a moment, standing up, his legs wobbling; he sat down with a thump on the grass. That seemed to suit him. If he hadn't been so filthy, the image of the child sitting in the long grass and daisies might have been idyllic.

We can't just walk away, Simon said. Anything could happen.

Anything could happen to us, too, Quentin said. Come on. His mother's going to come and find him.

Look at him, Simon said. What if he's been wandering around for days?

He'd be crying, Quentin said. Someone's looking after him. Just not very well. There's nothing we can do. Come on.

I'm not going, Simon said. You can't walk away from that.

Yes, I can, Quentin said. It's what we're going to do. Walk away. And in a minute someone will notice he's wandered off again and come and scoop him up.

If you walk away from this ... Simon said.

His sentence trailed off. He sounded uncertain. A future must be rising up before him in which he took the child himself, and walked in the other direction, back to his home; presented it to Mummie, his mummie, Linda; explained; explained again. Linda's head in her hands, her regretful stare laden with foreknowledge. And then what? The child's owner came in search of it, machete ready? Why had he said that – If you walk away from this – as if beginning an ultimatum or an undying moral truth? Quentin saw: he had started a sentence and realized, after six words, that he was saying a sentence written by someone else, in a student play he had been in. The new set of the shoulders told you that. If you walk away from this. He did not know how to return the sentence to the circumstances.

I feel terrible, Simon said in the end. The child had forgotten them; head down, he was poking his forefinger into the earth with delight, seeing how far it would go.

Everyone always feels terrible, Quentin said. If that's any consolation. About everything. You walk away from it, though. I don't know what the alternative to walking away is.

But this, Simon said. Just walking away and leaving him, not knowing he's safe.

Children are safer than you think, Quentin said, wishing that were true. He's nothing to us. We've got to get out of here before someone turns up blaming us for something.

I can't, Simon said. I just can't.

He knelt down, unhooking his rucksack and putting it on the ground. He unzipped the bag, and got out a little tuck box. Inside were the digestive sandwiches Linda had promised Quentin she'd make for her son – sad little circles of brown, encasing a square of yellow cheese. Simon held one out to the child. You could see what it cost him, and for a moment, with the child's attention on the earth, he wavered uncertainly; might have taken it back. Then the child raised his head. He grabbed it; stuffed it into his dirty mouth.

He's ravenous, Simon said.

Give him some water or he'll choke, Quentin said. Simon did so. He'll be okay now till someone comes looking for him.

I hope you're right, Simon said, putting his rucksack back on in the same sententious style. His jaw jutted; he tugged at the straps. He had settled on his action. They went on, leaving the child to his fate.

For a time they said nothing to each other. The signs of the town to their right were thinning. Quentin had never learnt to read a map and did not have one. He had gone from place to place guided by the satellite navigator or by the satellite navigator of others. The town was breaking up; the borders were going up. Soon you would know when you had passed out of one territory into another by the appearance of guards, gangs, warnings. When he had bought the house, the estate agent had taken him from property to property, trying each time to explain what each area was like, its associations and its flavour. Quentin had found this amusing, partly because the estate agent was not naturally articulate, and struggled to put words to what was clear in her mind, resorting to Nice and Lively and Attractive to euphemize what she could not say. It was also, at that remote time, a curiosity because on no level could a stranger distinguish a nice neighbourhood of bungalows from a lively one. They both appeared quiet, groomed, given to the cultivation of apple trees and clematis, clean. Perhaps she meant that a Black family lived in the lively neighbourhood. All that was sharpened and growing, and would go on growing in people's minds until it took on a reality. Quentin had no map and, after years of satnav, didn't think he could read one now there was nothing better, but it made no difference. All he had had to do was walk to the margin of the land and turn right, following the sea eastwards, on his left hand, until they reached what had once been Ramsgate. Before that, they would pass through one suburb after another, one territory before a new one made itself evident, where those dim flavours were enough to make a country, to drive the watchers to take a stance and tell the unfamiliar face in their lands to make a move. The borders would go up and the watchers would take control. And Simon, like the small child they had just walked away from, had been abandoned.

Quentin had never been so sure of anything. Linda had sent Simon off that morning with a clear farewell. Where she was going Quentin could not say. But she was leaving. Perhaps it was to a sister, a friend, an old boyfriend, or just to somewhere she had heard about. Linda had lived here all her life, and she would know that her bungalow on Savile Crescent would not shelter her if things went wrong. There were glass windows; there was a thin wooden fence. On the wooden fence, the side facing the pathway between the houses, impatient marks in white paint had sprouted overnight, this last two weeks. Three different symbols. What they indicated, nobody could say. Linda thought they were just trying to scare us. But who they were was unclear, and would stay unclear.

That morning, they had said goodbye, and Linda had hugged her son. Perhaps that was a normal gesture between them, but Quentin didn't think so; Simon had gone rigid, had retreated and given her a look. I'll see you around, Linda had said, perhaps mostly to Quentin. I don't know when I'll be back, Quentin said truthfully. Maybe when things improve. Yeah, Linda said. And you – she stepped forward and hugged her son again, perhaps with more intention to demonstrate something this time. I love him to bits, she said to Quentin, when the hug had run its course. Simon was inspecting her, his arms to one side, his madman's transparency of blue in the eyes shining with alarm, like carbuncles in the sun. I just love him to bits, she said again, and Simon dutifully echoed, as far as he could. I love you too, Mum, he said. And then that was it. Quentin was sure that was the last time either he or Simon would see Linda. What was the distinction between what Simon had said, I love you, which was a sentiment spoken in every language on earth since the human race had learnt to form sounds into meaning, and what Linda had said, I love you to bits, which was merely an idiom of surface enthusiasm and profound disengagement. I love you to bits, but I can't shop here any more since you put up that flag of a swastika. I love you to bits, but I've met a boy called Darren, and I'm moving out this afternoon. I love you to bits, because you're my pet hamster, and you won't live more than two years at best. Linda had said, I love him to bits. She had been wearing a clean blouse and clean trousers, astonishingly pressed and unworn. They must have been preserved at the back of the wardrobe for just such an occasion as this. Such an occasion: the saying goodbye to your only son, waiting till your kind neighbour has taken him out of sight, and getting into your car with the two inches of petrol in the tank, and driving to a safer place, on your own, with all your stores in the boot to bargain with. What that place was Quentin could not say; the farmhouse of a friend where you could see people coming a mile off, or the top flat in a secure block with a rooftop you could sit on and a stair that could be booby-trapped. A brother, a friend, a colleague, a lover lived in one of these places. Simon was doing her head in, as she had admitted, and her host would not take him. It was not important. Children were abandoned all the time; children abandoned their families all the time. It didn't matter. Quentin was on his way to his father, or that was his story. In fact, now he could see that he had abandoned his father long ago. If Scott was at home and would take him in, he would go no further. And Simon would be long disposed of before then.

They had been walking for three hours now. If Simon's watch was accurate, it was a bit after ten o'clock. The early mist had lifted off the sea and clarity and glitter had taken its place. There was a slight breeze behind them. Out to sea, an abandoned cargo ship shone orange, like a drawn line, and behind them a clueless queue of wind turbines, scattered in a haphazard way. Their blades were still turning, senselessly. Where was that electricity going? Perhaps his father had been right, and they were being turned by artificial means. Where, then, were they getting the electricity from? Was someone, after all, in charge, unseen?

I'm thirsty, Simon said. They hadn't spoken for some time. Simon had performed downcast after they had left the child digging with its paws in the sward.

Have some water, Quentin said.

I would, but I've run out, Simon said. I only brought a litre. More than that would be too heavy to carry, I thought. I've drunk it.

Well, that's tough, Quentin said. He would not offer him any of the litre-and-four-fifths left in his rucksack. If Simon had guzzled his store, that was his lookout.

A little later – they were approaching the big 1930s road-house pub that was said to have quite good meals, the Fox and Hounds – Simon said again, I'm thirsty. I'm honestly really thirsty.

Oh, God.

I just thought we'd be able to find some on the way. There's always water around.

I can't see how, Quentin said.

There must be some in there, in the pub, Simon said.

Have some sense, Quentin said. Look at it.

The Fox and Hounds, said to have good food, was a shell. The windows were all blackened with a weeks-old fire; the letters of the pub's name were stained with smoke and soot. There was nothing inside it, not even a bottle of water. It had been looted and destroyed. On the brick wall separating what had been garden and kiddies' playground from what had been pavement and road, a sign had been sprayed or painted. Quentin saw that it was the same sign that someone had slashed on Raine's fence, an equals sign with a line through it. Perhaps this was what was decreed for her. For a moment he felt the atrocious muscle memory that forced his hand towards the pocket where a phone, an internet signal, sweet scurrying Google ought to have lived, eager to explain what he was look-ing at. But all that was gone, and what was left was only the twitch of his hand in the direction of clearness and knowledge.

Yes, Simon said. It was an awful pub, anyway. Mummie would never go there. There was too much danger of running into Luke or one of his minions. You know he sells drugs, my brother? That's the nearest to us he comes, the back bar of that pub. Or used to come. There's another pub Mummie likes to go to instead. It's only three or four streets inside. She says it's a really old pub and the town's grown up around it. Do you know it?

What's it called?

The Whit Arms. Nobody goes there much but it's nice. Actually nobody much knows about it. It's in a strange place, houses all around it and a recreation ground in front. We could check that out. I bet they'll have gone for this one on the front but not that one.

I don't know, Quentin said. He wondered about venturing inland, into a mesh of streets he didn't know.

We can go in and just take a look and then out again, Simon said. If it looks off. I'm going to die if I don't get any water.

Just to look and then out again, Quentin said.

The sensation of leaving the open spaces of the grass topping the beach and venturing even three streets inland was of moving from one element into another. They turned their back on the sea, but walking past the black-burnt shell of the road-house pub into a stretch where houses stood blank and unpeopled on either side felt like the waters closing above their heads. For a moment Quentin felt physically small, encased, as if he had forgotten to take a deep breath before entering. There was no movement anywhere. The houses might have been abandoned. That was to reassure himself, however, and they might, too, be just now attracting attention. The houses had no front gardens. Their fronts abutted the pavement, and only by walking in the centre of the road could they keep a safe distance from where people might be concealing themselves for their own purposes.

What's that, Simon said, his voice lowered. Some way off, at the corner of a street, a dark movement, close to the ground. At first it could have been someone crawling, a small child again. Then it moved, a jerky buckling, and an abrupt cough of a noise. It was a dog, and at its first bark more dogs emerged from the traverse street, following their pack leader. They approached. There were twelve or thirteen of them, matted and dirty, and at the back one had stopped, curled up and gnawed his balding side with great force. The pack had been pets until a few weeks ago; they were not street dogs, but breeds said to be lovable, liberated from laps and sheepskin beds by the side of radiators. The leader, now standing staring at them with implacable concentration, was a black and tan dachshund, and by him was a matted schnauzer, its beard thick and clotted and tangled, like Rastafarian dreads; the rest were crossbreeds, bred for easy affection and now practised fighters, cockapoos, schnorgis, maltichon, shihtadors, laboratory inventions where the wolf was coming, late, to the surface. There was nothing to be scared of here. This was a pack liberated from a suburb of bungalows and small, tidy gardens. None of the dogs was more than two feet tall. They inspected these unknowns; in a moment they would surely trot up, their bright eyes shining, begging adorably for scraps and a tummy tickle. But they did not trot up. They stayed as they were, wary and scrupulous, assessing what their chances might be in every direction. One of them barked, near the back of the pack, out of bravado, before turning and scuttling off. The rest of the undecided pack paused. Simon bent and picked up a pebble from the gutter; he threw it with a crack at the leader. A chorus of barking asserted the dignity of the pack. But they ran. In another month they would not run.

Where's this pub, said Quentin. We shouldn't hang around.

It's just here, Simon said. Look, it's fine.

As Simon had told him, the pub was curiously situated, in a side-street between pairs of semi-detached houses. It was older than the suburb around it. Silence had returned; the commotion of the dog pack had not drawn anyone's attention. The pub was squat, white, its slate roof low, and an odd shape, lumpy with functional, rather than elegant, extensions; a toilet block had been necessary, and a kitchen pushed back into the yard. It had escaped notice by the looters and gangs; the windows were boarded up, but there was no painted symbol that could be seen.

We're not going to get in, Simon said.

Doesn't look like it, Quentin said. Give it a go.

But they went up to the door. There was a piece of paper pinned to it; someone had wanted to have it sealed in clear plastic, but, lacking the means, had settled for wrapping the notice in clingfilm. It could just about be read. We Did Not Close Then. And We Are Not Closing Now. We Carry On.

Yeah, Quentin said. Well.

Simon put his ungloved hand on the door handle, and twisted. Neither of them expected the door to open; Quentin had the impression of having jumped back in shock. The interior was quite dark; the windows had been efficiently boarded against the day. Whether it was more of an exposure to the unknown to go in or to retreat held them there for a moment, silhouetted against the bright day for anyone within.

Go in, Simon said. There's no one there.

How can I help you, gentlemen. A voice came from the dark, and a glint sparked from behind the bar.

I'm sorry, Quentin said. I didn't think there was anyone here.

We never closed then and we aren't closing now, the voice said. It had at first seemed like a woman's; now it started to have the faint worry of a light tenor. Only the customers need careful sifting. I know you, don't I?

I used to come here with my mother, Simon said. Before.

That's right, the voice said. Come in and shut the door. A nice lady. Always complimented us on our service, always had the whitebait. That's right. And we could do with a bit of light, maybe.

The landlord struck a match; he lit a candle on the bar, and the room was faintly illuminated. It had been a pub interior of the most ordinary country variety; wood pillars dividing up the bar, brass-handled beer pumps, dark glass-doored fridges holding bottles behind, and in the main room spindly dark wood tables and stools and the occasional sticky chair with arms, a dark red patterned carpet, and around the walls, hunting scenes and engravings, presumably of local countryside and historic houses, brass, too, the unused fire implements and horseshoes and minatory notices. Do Not Ask For Credit, one ran, Because A Punch In The Face Often Offends. They would have to offer credit now, or give it away, or demand the printed notes and coins that no one used or had; there was really no such thing as money any more. The landlord was alone; he wore a waxed cotton coat as if about to leave. Some effort had been made, but the white shirt that was tucked in had a thick tidemark of black around the collar. On the bar in front of him was a revolver, its handle towards him. His face was lined, his hair a shock of grey; his smell of neglect filled the room.

My wife had it, he said. And I had it. You might remember her. She was the motherly type, everyone always said, the motherly type of landlady. The motherly type of barmaid when I first met her, thirty years back, behind the bar of this pub as it happens. It was her old dad who had the licence. She caught it and I caught it, the beginning of what they're calling the fifth wave. And I got over it in a week, and her, it finished her off. Poor old Mary. Heart of gold.

We were only looking for some water, Simon said.

You're not from round here, the landlord said. Not a question.

We've walked about five miles, Quentin said. We're from the Savile estate. That's where we live.

Not from round here, the landlord said. No harm in that. I'll see what I can do. You know, you're the first people in five days to try to come in the pub. You're more polite than the last lot. I don't mind. You can have some water. I'd sell it to you, only what's the point.

He opened the dark fridge behind him and took out four small bottles of water.

That's still holding up, just about, he said. It's warm, though. The beer's finished, weeks ago. And the last lot that came in, they took what was left of the whisky and the gin and the vodka. The beer went first. We were running low when it all fell apart. The order wouldn't go through – the banks were down. You took from the suppliers, the breweries, and you distributed it to the eager punters. It worked like a dream until it stopped working. I had no idea how to fix it. I don't suppose they did either. Then Mary and me, we caught it. The staff didn't want to come in and we closed for ten days. I came back in – we don't live over the shop, or didn't, we used to live a mile off, nice house – came back in and the phones had gone, too. Electricity out; laptop just a piece of expensive metal. I went back up the coast and watched my wife die. Then I came back here. I think it's safer. Still providing a bit of a service, anyway. As you see.

Thanks, buddy, Quentin said.

I'd rather you didn't call me buddy, the landlord said, with a flourish of the old style.

Quentin gave an embarrassed tip of the head.

If you'd come a week ago, I could have cooked you something, he said. Even if it was eggs or out of a tin, whatever. Had an old Calor gas stove out the back. Finally ran out. Ran out of gas, I mean. Never mind. Things will come back at some point. I don't really know how bad things have got from the virus point of view. Been a while since we've heard from the government or the *News at Six*. It might all be getting back to normal. Somehow.

If I were you, Quentin said. I wouldn't stay here.

The landlord raised his head in the dark and the candlelight, a chiaroscuro skull. His eye sockets were deep, and his eyes a glitter in the dark wells of bone. At once there was a heavy noise from above, and another, and another, as something landed on and stomped over the roof. Some sort of chant came from the same direction; human, rhythmic, unrestrained in its joy.

They're having fun, the landlord said. The life-to-come boys. They do this sometimes. They must have seen you coming in. They think it scares me. Only – He laid his hand on the revolver on the bar. Was it real, or a replica? Had it been fired? Impossible to say, in the half-light, and it would be impossible, too, for the boys, coming with a swagger through the door, bearing, perhaps, their pointed sticks, their certainty of impunity. The revolver had power, and its power lay in its never having been fired. One day that power would leave it.

They don't scare me, the landlord said, quite calmly.

Oo-gher – oo-gher – oo-gher – oi – oi – oi – oi – the boys outside, squatting on the roof, appeared to say. Then a word. Paedo, one voice shouted, then again, Paedo, Paedo, Paedo, Paedo.

So long as they stick to that, I won't object, he went on. Sometimes they do it in the night. That's not so pleasant. It's right above your head. They know when they do it at three in the morning that's going to wake an old man up. But I lock the doors at night, the door to the outside and the door to the flat, and they haven't tried to come in through the roof yet. It's just making noise. That's all it is. You'll want to be on your way.

You ought to come with us, Simon said.

Don't be stupid, the landlord said, with an abrupt and incontrovertible snarl. Come with you where? And leave the business to, what, that lot? I'm staying here. On your way.

It seemed reckless to leave the pub while the invaders plunged and jousted on the roof. The thunderous row hardly made the landlord blink, but he had heard it before, had known it not come to anything. Or they could wait until it stopped, and the boys, whoever they were, had moved on. Wait until dark, and what dark might bring. The dogs; the glitter of flaming torches; a crucifixion of a small being, down there where a housewife had, that morning, had to take a shit. They should go, and take their chance. Simon could follow, or he could stay.

Come on then, Quentin said, and opened the door. He walked briskly into the sun, not looking back. The noise behind escalated. Something was thrown. There was Simon, hurrying into his back, pushing and, what Quentin had determined not to do, breaking into a run. A thrown slate landed to their side, shattering on the road. So they were getting through the roof. They could come through the door in daylight if they chose. But they would come through the roof, at three in the morning. That was their choice. It wouldn't be long for the landlord and his replica revolver now. The noise was behind them, but static, profane, wordless, obscene, and the pack of dogs was answering it. They were staying where they were, squatting above their prey. He would scare them off; and then he would not scare them off. Paedo, the voices went on, Paedo, Paedo, Paedo.

Before Quentin knew it they were back in the open, at the top of the shingle slope, released from the enclosed medium of streets. Oh, houses, how I hate you all, he said again to himself. The sea was as it had always been.

Did you see, Simon said.

But Quentin had not. He had walked forward indifferently and with speed, not looking back or engaging with the mob on the roof.

One of them – Simon said. He was wearing a policeman's jacket and helmet. There were three of them. On the roof. One of them, he was a policeman.

I don't believe it, Quentin said.

It had been good, that evening. The last evening of its kind. Something had been different about it, or was that just knowing what he now knew? Scott was a good, funny person. He was going to do well. He wrote music for movies – he'd done well writing music for TV ads straight out of college, Brick Builds You Up was his and who could see a Brick bar in the newsagent without thinking of that encouraging four-note tune? Now he was getting commissions for whole films.

It's not hard, these days, he said, his head down, chopping onions in Quentin's kitchen. The brief basically just said, Make it like the music for Dunkirk. Menacing growl for ninety minutes. They want it all in place for when restrictions lift and they can start filming again with a crew and actors. It's all electronic from my side. I'm doing the whole lot in the shed in the garden in Kentish Town and they can decide later if they'd prefer an orchestra. I don't know what happened to war movies. Music for war movies, I mean. It must have been more work writing *633 Squadron*.

What's that?

Oh, come on, you know *633 Squadron*. Sixties movie. Famous tune. Scott sang a little, with gusto – he sang in tune, but the voice was shot and gravelly.

Maybe, Quentin said after a bit.

Anyway, they don't want that, Scott said. They just want a stretch of material going …

He made an extraordinary noise, ascending in a low growl from a deep point, a single note, climbing in degrees like a bus going up a hill. Quentin watched him singing with his head back; he could have watched him all day, he reckoned. He ran out of breath.

The good thing is when they say, It needs another fifteen seconds here, or We're cutting this by a minute. It's no trouble, you just measure it out like a length of schmutter, whatever the customer desires. Ron Goodwin couldn't have done that, with his four four-bar phrases, take one, take the lot. Am I getting professional?

No, no. Who's Ron – Ron –

Goodwin. Wrote the mu for *633 Squadron*. Still I'll get an Oscar for this crap – it's got prestige written all over it. Want to be my date? Look good in a tux, don't we?

Scott had said it lightly, but the Oscars had not happened for three years now, and this film wouldn't be released for another two. Was that a promise, or an offer that would never be redeemed?

Hey, Scott said. He was in a good mood, full of bounce, and when he turned round his eyes danced over Quentin in his white bathrobe out of the shower; he'd been like this in the past, after he'd fucked and been fucked. There was a disaster. I forgot to say. I was going to get cheese. I just thought – yeah, cheese. Then, this is like an hour ago, I'm in Waitrose, I turn down the cheese aisle and it's empty. Nothing. The whole lot's gone, apart from this kind of weird orange stuff and something in a tube and something I actually considered getting, Cheddar flavoured with, I don't know, banana or turmeric berries or chilli or something. What's going on?

Don't ask me, ask Waitrose, Quentin said.

No cheese, Scott said. Can you believe it.

Can live without it.

Brexit.

That one's wearing a bit thin, Quentin said.

Yeah, Scott said. He lit the gas, placed the frying pan on it, poured a swipe of olive oil into it, lifted the chopping board and swept the sliced onion in. After a couple of moments it began its sibilant cook. The side of salmon, too big for two, gleamed in its bowl of Sichuan oils and wine, of peppers and pickles, waiting its turn.

(Thinking about it now, the single striking thing: all that was gone, from gas to oil to fish to pickles, used up, irreplaceable as cheese. Scott too.)

He went on for a while, then lowered the heat.

Quent, he said.

Yeah, Quentin said.

Scott turned round. He was about to say something. The shine in his eyes had altered in some way; he was just looking at Quentin, about to say something he had prepared and thought over.

Doesn't matter, he said brightly. Just wanted to say Quent.

No one's ever called me Quent.

Well, I'll always remember I was the first, Scott said. And the evening went its way, the last evening there was ever to be. He was certain that Scott had been about to say something momentous, something he had prepared and decided on as he drove over, or perhaps in the days preceding. And it was impossible to know what Scott's sentence would have been. You could pretend that you knew the inside of people's heads, that you could roam around gathering the thoughts of others as a bad novel could pop inside the heads of one character after another, saving time and explaining what everyone felt. But in reality he could look at Scott and determine only his most immediate desires, to get hold of Quentin, to leave because he was bored, to fall asleep, and perhaps that was it. Scott's surface: the look on his face, the way he held his arms, the distance between his feet, the way he now shook his salt-encrusted hands with professional confidence, like a big horse drying his mane after a splash of water; that surface was all you had to go on. When Scott had turned away from the hissing onions and looked with an expression of real kindness at Quentin in his bathrobe, it could have meant any number of things. That was what Quentin had felt at the time, without paying much attention, because in a moment Scott would speak and clear up the vagueness. But Scott had not said anything; he had stepped back from what he was about to say. In the ten weeks since, Quentin had gone over that look, and had tried to determine what had been behind that kindly but almost apologetic gaze, glistening only with the tears of an onion-chopper, and he thought it might have meant one of two things. Scott might have been about to say that he and Quentin were doing all right – did Quent want to make a thing of it? It was too early to talk about moving in, but that would have been a first step. Or there was the other thing. Scott could have been about to say something final, that it had been fun and Quent was a great guy, but maybe the time had come. There were two things Scott could have said there, only one of which had ever been said to Quentin. The first was: I've met this other guy I really like. The other one – words Quentin had only ever heard in movies Scott wrote the music to, for money – was the old one. I love you.

Anyway, it had not been said. They had fucked again in the morning; there had been a sort of breakfast, made up of two Bloody Marys each and the last six oysters, three each. Scott had got into his car and driven off, vaguely saying he'd have to remember to fill up tomorrow. And that evening he had gone to switch the light on, and the electricity was off, and his phone was out of battery. And that was the last of Scott.

What does that mean, Simon said. They had been walking in silence for an hour after leaving the pub. The sea had continued on their left; the heights had shrunk, and they were now walking on the same level as the sea. They had passed through a desolate town, all the shop fronts facing the beach smashed and emptied, many of them burnt. A curious tower like a removed church spire still stood on the parade. There were no people to be seen or heard at all. At one point they had seen a high-stepping graceful deer going through the streets, careless of its likely fate. Some rage had swept through this town and sent a warning to anyone thinking of setting up some means of protection. They had been glad to leave that place, in silence, and not met with anything. Now they had approached some ruin, a stone tower and some broken-down stone walls. On the walls somebody had sprayed a sentence in purple paint, and they stood and read it together.

THE LIFE TO COME IS NOT THE LIFE THAT WAS.

Before the first word and after the last word was the same symbol they had seen outside their own houses, an ineptly drawn clockwise spiral. What it meant was no clearer to Quentin than it had ever been. The life to come: he had heard that somewhere before, and recently.

I can't believe they did that, Simon said. They'll be furious when they see their fort's been sprayed on.

What is it?

Don't you know the Roman fort? It's been here for ever – well since the Romans, I suppose. No. If you didn't go to school round here, then probably not. But if you did, you got to know it quite well. It's very boring really, just a pile of old stones the Romans put up to watch out to sea. We got taken here all the time, every year almost. Then we had to do a project about it usually, the Romans and what they were doing here and how they built and all that. They invented central heating, did you know? Well, sort of.

I've never been this way, Quentin said. Or only in a car.

The life to come, Simon said.

Let's not hang around, Quentin said.

Look, Simon said.

Behind them, hastening, a figure that seemed to be running with great expense of energy to not much purpose, like a bundle of washing being tossed around by a strong wind. There did not seem to be much threat to it, and Simon and Quentin waited. In a few minutes it became clear that it was the man they had left behind, the landlord of the Whit Arms. He was wearing what he had been wearing, the waxed cotton jacket and the white shirt with the black ring of dirt around the collar. Now he had been bloodied. Dried blood ran from his nose, and the left side of his face was beginning to develop a bruise, a black eye. He looked wild.

They came through the roof, he said. His voice panted; there was something in his mouth that made him speak thickly. He spat and said it again.

You had to get out, Quentin said.

Where to, the man said. There was nothing to be said to that. Paedo with your paedo friends.

Is that what they said?

Paedo with your paedo friends, he said again. They came through the roof. There's nothing you can do if they're going to come through the roof.

Are you going to your house, Simon said.

How do you know about my house, the man said. How do you know?

You told us, Quentin said. Simon looked both shocked and frightened, as if the man's raised voice might turn into the same violence he had been through. You told us you'd got a house a mile up the road as well as the flat above the pub. The pub was going to be safer, you thought.

Yeah, the man said. I told you. I'd forgotten. It's gone, though, that house. They broke in and when they were done it looked like they'd smashed it up and set it on fire for the fun of it. All my girl Mary's pretty things. I hadn't seen what they'd done until just now and I walked straight on. I didn't know what they were, if they were still about. It's all gone.

He said the last three words again with terrible emphasis, as if saying it would take the harm out of it. Then he seemed to grow peaceful. He sat. Time passed.

You're not in with the life-to-come boys, he said. You didn't write that. That's a Roman fort, you know. They can't burn that down. That's always been there, long as I remember.

We used to come here on school trips, Simon said. I was just saying. He sat, too.

Long as I remember that's been here, the man said. You were supposed to come here and look out to sea with your girl. This would have been in the eighties. I thought I was supposed to, so I said to Mary on her day off, Come on, let's walk up to the Roman fort. And she went along with it, and she was waiting for me in this red coat she really loved at the time, cherry red it was called, waiting in the pub car park. We walked along the coast until we got here – she made me laugh, that Mary, always did. And then we got here and sat down and she said, I'm cold, darling, give us a cuddle, and I gave her a cuddle. I'd been worrying about something stupid, that there'd be other people at the Roman fort, having a kiss and a cuddle, that it would look like everyone only came here for one purpose, but there was only us there and she'd have liked it anyway.

Everyone likes a kiss and a cuddle, Quentin said. He tried to keep the impatience out of his voice. But the man hardly heard him.

We were sitting there, there, just there, he said. That was the first time, the first place we ever had a kiss. After a bit she said to me, Interested in old ruins, then, are you? And I thought she couldn't mean her because she was younger than me, I didn't know what she meant, so I said, No, no. To be on the safe side. And she said, I'm bloody freezing, so let's get out of here and back to your mum's house. I must have mentioned to her at some point that my mum was out. And we went back to my mum's house and in a manner of speaking we never left each other ever again, and we never come back here to the Roman fort in any case. We never needed to. It's all that matters, love, that's all there is. And you're inside it or you're outside it. You never wrote that, did you?

No, Quentin said. If he talked calmly and slowly, here at the point where the Romans had built, where they had looked out and seen what he now saw, the cold glitter of sea going for miles and miles, then perhaps the wildness would leave this man. Perhaps he would soon return to the superior worldliness he had displayed behind his bar. Perhaps he would return to the language he knew how to use, and not betray his Kentish childhood by saying, We never come back here. Perhaps; and perhaps that was gone for ever. We never wrote that. Who are they? The life-to-come boys?

They come through the roof, didn't they, the landlord said.

You had a gun, Simon said, his voice rising.

They took that, didn't they, the landlord said. We'll be back with this, they go. Then they're off. We'll have some fun, won't we, Dave, they say. My name's not even Dave. First this, the handle of the gun did this, whop, and I'm down, down on the floor. Then they're off. Paedo with your paedo friends. Paedo with your paedo friends. I had to get out of there.

Where are you going, Quentin said. The man got to his feet.

You said, the landlord said. He said. He said you could take me along with you. I said no but I fear I may have spoken too hastily. The situation has altered somewhat. As you see.

The man smiled, or tried to. His lip was split and bleeding; the ruin of his mouth was not to be inspected closely.

We can't do that, Quentin said. We've kept out of trouble quite well till now.

And I'll be out of trouble if I'm with you, the landlord said.

Simon had stood up. He was clearly one of those people who found physical damage impossible to be near. This was Quentin's to solve.

You can't, Quentin said. You'll have to look after yourself.

Just for a few miles, the landlord said. I'll be no trouble.

No, Quentin said. Fuck off.

If they come for me, the landlord said.

Yeah, Quentin said.

If they come for me they'll come for me. You want that on your conscience, do you?

Fuck off, Quentin said.

I gave you, the man said. I gave you, I didn't even charge you, I gave you –

A bottle of water, Quentin said. Now fuck off. Go on. Fuck off.

The landlord came closer – much closer than the ten-feet distance, an abject look in his bloodied eyes, almost cringing. Quentin did what he had only done once or twice before. He drew back a fist and punched the man, hard. The landlord staggered back, making a small cry. There was no further discussion. He turned and ran, hugging himself, into the world of houses and bungalows, sheds and hiding places, fences and ambushes, avenues and crescents and closes, a world of enclosure and violence and the sealess, the skyless, the airless.

Come on, Quentin said.

They'll kill him when they find him, Simon said. You punched him.

Yeah, Quentin said. Needed to be done. Come on.

THE LIFE TO COME IS NOT THE LIFE THAT WAS.

How could you, Simon said.

It had to be done, Quentin said. Now fuck off or come along.

I can't believe –

Fuck off, then.

It's over, Simon said. My life. It's fucking over.

He had fallen to his knees in the middle of the road.

I don't care, Quentin said. I'm leaving you. I can't be doing with this drama. I just need to get to Ramsgate.

He did not move, however. His knuckles hurt. He must have hit bone when he struck the landlord, and he did not know what it was like to punch another man. He told Simon to get up, quite roughly; he walked four steps before stopping in an irresolute way.

It's true, Simon said. My life's over. I never managed to have one. I never came close to love and now I never will.

Oh, for fuck's sake.

Simon didn't move. Quentin waited. He thought of walking away. Then it was as if something more were called for. He walked back; he sank to his haunches.

You'll meet someone, Quentin said. There was something so kindly and close about talking to anyone, even Simon, within two feet of the ground. You always think it'll never happen and then one day it just happens.

It won't, Simon said. He beat his limp hands on the ground, ineffective, but full of rage. How do you meet people? How do you meet men? On apps. Don't exist. In bars. Don't exist. Coming close to people in the street, on Matchcombe beach after midnight, don't exist, don't exist, don't exist. You'll never meet anyone ever again. Is there love or is there not love? It doesn't matter. I am always going to be outside love. I might as well be dead. And Mummie's gone. I know she has.

Why do you think that, Quentin said, getting up.

She's definitely gone. You know she has.

How should I know that.

She has. You know something. Those biscuits she gave me. Just biscuits with a bit of old cheese. That was the last food in the kitchen, the last food she'd got. And I knew I shouldn't ask it but this morning I asked it anyway. I said, What are you going to do for food. And she said, Oh, I'll be all right. She was wearing some clothes she's not worn for ages, too.

Just fucking get up.

Get up in a moment.

Get up now.

All right. I'm getting up, look, I'm getting up. I don't know where she's going but she's gone.

Linda wouldn't just leave you like that.

It's okay, Simon said. I'll find Luke and then I'll be all right. Luke isn't going without, I know that much. He'll always land on his feet. I'll be all right if I get there. I'm the opposite. I'll always land – What's the opposite of someone who always lands on his feet?

Someone who never lands on his feet.

That's rubbish, Simon said.

All right, Quentin said. You know what the opposite is? Someone who no one would miss.

Simon looked away. They went on walking.

I always liked these houses, he said, after a few minutes. They were passing a series of solid detached houses, gated and boarded. I always said to my mum that one day when I'm a famous actor I'll buy one of these, five or six bedrooms and a garden with a gardener to take care of it, and she says, my mum always says, Oh, yeah, that'll be nice, as if I hadn't said anything at all ... Nobody will miss me. Is that what you think?

That's not what I said.

That's what you said. It's over for me. You're right, really.

Forget it.

There's nobody there who I'm never going to – How is anyone going to meet anyone now? How am I going to meet anyone?

Yeah. You have a point.

There's just no way. You can't come close to someone you don't know and you can't meet anyone and nobody you do know will do and –

You're not making any sense.

I just want some love in my life, said Simon.

Quentin understood what he was saying, but what he was saying was pathetic.

You got your timing right, Simon said. You've got a boyfriend. You know when you told me you were gay and I went, No way, I don't believe it? I was pretending. Of course I knew you were gay. Everyone knows you're gay. That ginger bloke who comes round, the one in the vest, every Saturday. Your boyfriend. Mr and Mrs Davies used to call you the bummers, not when I was in the room, but just to my mum and I heard them. They thought it was really funny, the big muscly bummer and his muscly ginger boyfriend.

I don't even know who Mr and Mrs Davies are.

They live opposite, the house with the cherry tree in the front garden and the blue Vauxhall Astra in the drive, or used to be. Everyone knows. It's just that you don't think they do. But even someone like you's got your boyfriend and I'm never going to meet anyone. It's all over and it never started for me.

Don't be so stupid, Quentin said. People find each other. You'll probably do better now that –

He held back. It was not a kind thing, what he was about to say.

What.

Nothing.

Now that there's not so much choice. That's what you meant.

That was what Quentin meant, but he adjusted the pack on his back and went on walking. Simon carried on talking. It was not worth listening to and Quentin did not listen. Simon was describing his future, of shivering in the corners of rooms, of his reliance on his brother's ability to inflict terror. Luke would have his fiefdom and his satraps; Simon would be safe if he could get to his brother. Safe and despised. Where would love be in this scenario? Tossed to him with contempt, like the carcass of a fish to a cat, which could crunch it. Or not at all.

He went on, Simon did, and in time he turned to the injustice of Quentin, the luck of him, dull and banal and unoriginal, the look of ten thousand others, interchangeable, and the same mind and thoughts as a million, and getting laid. It was something Simon must have devoted time to thinking over, and to him, Quentin was a prodigy of availability: no rejection had ever come Quentin's way and no blankness of response. He just had to reach out to be gratified. Quentin could see that there was no sex as gymnastically satisfying as the sex he performed in Simon's head. He let Simon go on talking, his penetrating voice like an insistent high clarinet, piping in the wind. I know it's just that I'm scared, Simon went on, I'm scared because of what a stranger might do to you, these days. They really might. Those people on the roof. Electricity stops and food delivery breaks down and you see what the human race is like.

It was lucky for the human race that none of it would have to listen to Simon for very much longer, Quentin said to himself.

Finally the complaint wound down.

Are you finished, Quentin said.

Simon shook his head. It perhaps meant that he was finished.

It's hot, Quentin said. He had thought about saying this. Maybe the time had come to say it, and for him to go on. I want to have a swim. Do you want to?

I can't swim, Simon said.

OK, Quentin said. Will you mind my clothes and stuff? I'll just be ten minutes. I didn't get my swim this morning.

Together they made their way across the shingle towards the sea. At one point Simon made a noise, a small shriek, which he converted into a cartoon noise of Whoops, falling on a falling stone. Quentin caught him; gallantly took his arm. There was nobody around. The cry of hungry seagulls filled the air, like the song of the sea, three notes wide. All this long, hungry day Quentin had carried out the instruction that he had once heard a depressive give to save himself from the worst fit. Don't think about the past; don't think about the future. What lay ahead of him and what surrounded him was what people could do, and what people would do. He felt he owed it to himself to close his mind against those future acts of darkness, crowding in on him, howling on the roof of any silenced refuge. By now Linda was gone, untraceable, banging on a stranger's door; now the landlord was wandering the streets in search of a refuge he would never find; now his little bungalow was looted and destroyed; now Raine was raped and dead, lying on her back in the front room with the windows smashed; now Buckley her dog hung crucified on the beach, his dark head dangling, his dear pink tongue lolling above the gashed throat. Now that small child was dead. Who knew how. On the wall outside Quentin's house some man was painting what he knew was the slogan Luke believed in, the proverb of the religion Luke might have founded. THE LIFE TO COME IS NOT THE LIFE THAT WAS. He thought of none of that. Simon sat down at the edge of the sea, looking outwards with trust. Quentin allowed the knowledge to flood in of what he had the night before permitted himself to do: he bent and he kissed Simon, tenderly, softly, as if he meant it. Simon did not mean it: he tightened and made a small noise in his throat. At first he pulled away; then, requiring himself to accept what he knew he wanted, he kissed back. The taste of Simon, his unbrushed teeth, the bad smell of his breath, the overlay of the last of the cheese he had eaten an hour before, all this made an interesting experience to Quentin, as he had known it would. He had thought about all of this. He detached.

I hadn't thought, Simon said. He moved his hands over his own face, an unusual gesture; he seemed to be feeling and assessing something. Then it was clear. This had hardly ever happened before, and Simon, who wanted to be an actor in a world of one-man shows with no chance of an audience, was trying to find out what a man's face was like when, without any hope or expectation, it has just been kissed by another man, one he has longed for.

It doesn't matter, Quentin said, dropping his rucksack behind him on the shingle. I want my swim.

He had thought he would do it before, but now he thought he would swim first. He tore Scott's T-shirt over his head, kicking his silver Onitsuka Tigers from his feet, peeling the socks off quickly. He undid the belt and undid the jeans; they were still tight, and as he pulled them off, he heard Scott's amused voice asking if he often went commando in other people's trousers. Just today, Scott, he would have said if he were here. He didn't look at Simon's reaction to his taking his clothes off. The clothes that Scott owned. He knew what the reaction would be; shy and averting. It didn't matter any more. He waded out; the water was still cold, and when it was up to his thighs, he leapt forward in a dive. The splash swallowed itself in a kind of gulp as he fell underwater into the veil of murk. THE LIFE TO COME IS NOT THE LIFE THAT WAS. He found himself in that new medium, a new life. If he succeeded in staying down here in this different element, transformed, growing gills, like a hero under a spell, the sounds of other beings would come to him in ways he could not predict. The crowds of whales calling across untroubled oceans with their fat melisma would call to him, too, and nearer, the castanetting crabs, dancing to seduce each other, beating on their armour, the gulps and yodels of plunging seals, the crackle of shoals of herring turning in their hundreds in terror, plunging for the cold depths between landmasses. He would stay down here as his body changed and he would come to hear them all. He continued, descending by force in the cold obscurity, his head down, as if by pushing himself further into the other element, he could himself bring about the transformation so many tellers had put into their stories. *And then the prince began to breathe, and the sea above his head was like a country breeze to him, and he felt his body stretch and change and to move in different ways ...* His vision was blurred but his touch was strong. He felt an iron bar or pole embedded in the bed of the sea between rocks, and he clung to it. He brought his knees up to his chest and swayed there for a moment, like a lily. His breath held; he could always hold his breath for a full minute, perhaps more, he knew that, and he held on, distant from the world behind and above, oblivious of it, floating in the being here and being now and knowing he would go, when the time came, forwards and downwards, never to return to that renounced element of air and stone and built things.

Matter intruded. His chest blazed inside. He let go and rocketed upwards. He had been ten feet deep, and his head and shoulders erupted into the air like a bomb. He took a big sobbing breath and leapt into what he did best, the butterfly stroke, churning up the sea. Behind him a voice was calling. He could not hear what it was saying, and he would not stop to listen. He flung himself at the water's surface and he flung himself from the water into the air. The sting of the splash on his chest each time he fell back down was a joy to him. He went on. After some time he saw that the edge of the land, which had been behind him, was now swinging towards him. He must have gone in a circle. He slowed and went into a different stroke, making for the shore where he had something to do.

I was worried for a moment there, the boy on the beach said.

Quentin was upright on the stony beach. He shook himself like a dog, splattering the boy with seawater. He picked a strand of seaweed from his thigh. The boy was fixing his full attention on Quentin's head, refusing to look downwards. To do what he wanted, to inspect and examine every bit of Quentin bare, and to be seen to be looking at the body before him, would be to carry out a ceremony of intimacy from which there would be no returning. Quentin had been inspected in such a way before, and had inspected others. Such a gaze was a commitment, and the boy shrank from that.

You're a good swimmer, the boy said. I was frightened for a minute, you were underwater so long. I thought you'd drowned! I didn't know what I'd do. I can't swim, I couldn't have saved you.

You'd have got up and carried on, Quentin thought. There isn't an alternative any more, no one to report the dead to, no one to investigate the facts, no consequences to follow. He said none of this. He stretched.

That splashing stroke, the boy said. Butterfly. You've got to be a good swimmer before they let you do that at all. Isn't it exhausting? It looks exhausting. I could never do that. Look at your muscles!

A flick of the eyes downwards. What was it he feared in making that downwards look? The silence was absolute. If there was any human being within a mile, they would not emerge and would not show themselves. What had kept men from themselves and the acts they dreamt of was gone now, the windows smashed, the interiors looted, the possibilities of exchange destroyed, the guardians of safety let loose to jump and hammer joyfully, their chests bared, on the roofs of strangers. Out there, people were starting to exult in the possibility that anything, now, could be done. The life to come is not the life that was. It was time to go.

Quentin went to his bag, carefully putting aside what he had been wearing, Scott's trousers and T-shirt. Inside the bag were his own clothes. He did not dress. His movements had been slow and leisurely; now they grew fast. He pulled out the kitchen knife from the side where it lay safe. He turned and struck at the boy. A sound came from the boy as he struck. The knife Quentin gripped went through the gap between collar bone and shoulder bone, plunging deep into the soft flesh. There was blood and the sound of a man who has been punched hard. He did it again, this time into the boy's chest, and again, and again. The feel of knife into living flesh was what he had thought it would be. It was the fast movement of metal in air, and then the sensation of meeting with animal flesh, and going on moving, with insistence. He did it again. He thought he would probably always remember this as long as he was here to remember it.

After a time, the thing was done. The world was just the same as it had been. It was empty, with one new thing in it. He left it where it was, moving his bag and clothes a few feet to the side to keep them clean. He walked into the sea, and again swam for five minutes. When he came out he still had the knife in his hand and it was clean. When he had thought about all this he had planned to throw the knife into the sea to be swept away. But he thought he would keep it. He left the thing where it was. The mother was gone; the brother had heard nothing from them for weeks. Nobody would miss it and nobody was there to insist on the consequences of what Quentin had just done. He dressed, taking his time, putting Scott's clothes in the rucksack along with the knife. Then he climbed the shingle beach and turned to the left, walking confidently. After a mile or two he put his sunglasses back on. He was probably only an hour or two from Ramsgate.

Once he had asked his father what the worst thing he had ever done had been. He had been on the verge of asking what the thing was he was most ashamed of; then he thought he would add a touch of objectivity to the question. It had been on that last trip to the garden centre. The dahlia they had taken, which they should have paid ten pounds for, was on the back seat of Quentin's car and had inspired the question.

Punched someone, his father said, without hesitation. Well. I didn't punch him. I pushed him and he fell over.

I thought you were going to say, Quentin said.

Say what.

Something about sleeping with people when you're married to other people.

That's not that bad, his father said. That's all part of life's rich tapestry. People always understand in the end. Your generation. Christ.

You pushed someone, Quentin said.

Yeah, his father said. This is back in the 1970s. At school, in fact. There was an art mistress who started this art group for anyone who wanted to join. And I joined because, to be honest, there was another reason. I wasn't so mad keen on art, but this girl, there was this girl. Very sincere, very serious, beautiful girl, loved to paint. Never paid me any attention so I joined the art group she was in. It went on for a few months. Happened on a Thursday afternoon after school. Then one day we went to the art room as usual and another teacher came in and said the art mistress in charge couldn't be there so it was cancelled. Everyone went home. Then the next week the same thing happened – cancelled. The third week the same thing. We're in the art room. I said, Christ, that fucking woman – can't be bothered, something more interesting's come up, to that effect. There's this other kid in the group, supposed to be talented. The girl I like was all over him. He's normally quite shy but he tells me to shut up, she's got a reason she can't make it. So I said, Bollocks, she's just an idle cow, and the conversation between the two of us got a bit heated. In the end he said that he happened to know that her husband's in the last stages of some cancer or other and hasn't got long, so she's spending all her time with him at the moment. Well, how the hell was I supposed to know? So it gets a bit more heated.

Wait a minute, Quentin said. The argument went on after that?

Little shit, his father said. Of course it went on. In the end I told him to fuck off and gave him a push and he fell over. That's probably the worst thing I ever did.

What happened?

Got into school the next day and there's a letter on my desk signed by all the kids in the art group saying that the kid I punched won't stay in the art group if I'm going to be in it. So they want me to stop coming. The girl I liked signed it too.

What happened to the art mistress's husband?

Died. I suppose he died. I don't know when, though. Probably when they said he would, within a few weeks. So I stopped going and then I went to dental school and became a dentist and never saw any of them ever again. It doesn't sound that bad now I tell it properly.

That was the worst thing you ever did, Quentin had said.

And now he carried on walking eastwards, the sea on his left and Ramsgate ahead of him. The steady rhythm of his feet tramping in the long silence of the empty towns was lulling. Ahead of him was a town with his father in it, cowering in a flat above his ransacked dental practice, spooning cold beans from a tin. In it, too, was Scott, in his cottage, who Quentin loved. As soon as he got there they would go over the house and make it as secure as it could be. They might not shiver in hiding; they might paint a warning on the front of the cottage and live as they chose. THE LIFE TO COME MEETS AN ARMED RESPONSE. That might do it if they could find any paint. The town was ruled by someone like Luke, with his satraps and underlings and the awed unquestioning devotion he was held in. Perhaps even by Luke himself, demanding the sorts of ritual statements and abasements that started as a play-ground game and ended as a religion. Quentin and Scott would make themselves safe against that. They would barricade the windows; they would do together whatever needed to be done. Quentin went on walking in the direction of Scott's unquestioning embrace, springing with a new energy. The oceans lay to his left. The sun was some way from setting still. It hung in the sky like a lantern. Far out to sea, the wind turbines glittered and turned, inscribing their traceless patterns on the flat blank surface of the oblong sky, maintaining their meaningless spectacle, waiting for someone who knew how to read it.

FOUR

ENTRELACEMENT

The dining room was to be cleaned and tidied, and prepared for supper every day by six o'clock. It was William's job. Not everybody had a dining room in his house. The dining room had a cherry-wood table in it, and around it six cherry-wood chairs, each with a square cushion of yellow velvet. William and his mother and father did not eat breakfast or lunch in the dining room, but in the kitchen at the pine table. During the day William's father worked in the study upstairs; his mother worked in the sitting room, on the new desk they had bought and placed in the alcove. William had his school classes in the dining room, and was allowed to do his homework on the dining table, with a large cork mat between the pad and the polished table surface, in case he damaged it.

That was what his mother said. William would not damage the surface of the table. It was his job to take care of it and he did take care of it.

His father and his mother were allowed to keep the papers and documents they were working from on their desks from one day to the next. His mother was neat with her papers, because the sitting room was also the family room; his father was less so, even leaving documents and books about the law in piles at his feet. But that was because the study was his room, and William did not often go into it.

Allowed by whom.

In the dining room, there was also a sideboard of dark wood. The wood came from Africa and the sideboard came from Great-grandfather's house in Lagos. William did not know what the wood was and nobody knew. When he was little, the picture above the sideboard was a photograph of his mother and father and him. One day it had been replaced by a painting of a mountain and a lake, an old-fashioned painting, and six photographs of him, his mother and father, grandfather and grandmother and the aunts and cousins; they were placed in matching silver frames in a group on top of the sideboard. Immediately William had seen that the silver frames being uniform showed that they had all been bought at the same time. If it was up to him the frames would have been different and different sizes, and people would have seen that Grandfather deserved his own frame and at another time William had deserved a different one.

In the corner of the room was an armchair covered in blue and brown flowered material, like canvas, and scratchy to sit on. The armchair had been bought as his father's Christmas present by his mother two Christmases ago. It had not been a surprise for him. William and his mother had gone to Peter Jones and chosen an armchair. But then when Christmas came, it was a different armchair. His mother had explained that she had gone with his father to make sure that he would like his present and his father had chosen a different armchair.

The other armchair had been left to its fate, first excited about being taken home, then left in the wall-less unloved spaces of Peter Jones, told it was not wanted any more.

Nobody had ever sat in the armchair in the corner of the dining room, as far as William could remember. Only when the dining room had been assigned to him to do his school-work and homework in did he take to sitting in it sometimes.

He sat in it to read books. In it, he had read *The Observer's Book of Trees*, *Jane Eyre*, *Nineteen Eighty-Four*, *Augustus Carp*, volumes thirteen and fourteen of the *Children's Britannica* from the first to the last page, and a book about Frank Whittle, who invented the jet engine, and a book about Marie Curie, who invented radioactivity. That was in the last month. Discovered radioactivity. William kept a notebook where he set down the books he had read when he had finished them and gave them stars out of ten. *Jane Eyre* was the first book he had read that he had given ten stars to. It was the best book he had ever read and he did not know whom he could share that with. It would be like crying in school.

There was still homework and schoolwork, although everything now was homework. *Work* ... at *Home* ... The laptop was on the table between breakfast and five o'clock, and if you were careful you could read a book to the side without anyone noticing when the work was boring and easy so that even Saffron Hill-Ngumbe could manage to do it.

William was allowed by his father and his mother to have his school classes in the dining room and to do his homework on the table, but he was not allowed to keep his homework on the table from one day to the next. He started at eight thirty after breakfast; at ten thirty he had a break with his mother, and they walked outside to the end of the street or around the garden. Lunch was at one, and for it, his father came downstairs into the kitchen. He always asked William what he had learnt that morning, which was sometimes hard to explain. If the lesson had been geared towards what Saffron Hill-Ngumbe and that lot could understand, his father would have been incredulous, like being told he had been learning to say the alphabet or what a primary colour was. The afternoon was also broken up by twenty minutes with his mother, when she often wanted a cup of coffee to keep her on her toes. At five, the day's work came to an end, and it was William's job to tidy the dining room and to set the table for dinner.

Once a fortnight he did his favourite job, which was to wax the cherry-wood table. He took everything off the dining table, and wiped it carefully with a dry cloth. He brought out two more cloths, the first, red, to apply the wax, the second, which was blue, to buff the table. First he opened the tin of wax, which he had brought from the cupboard under the kitchen sink at lunchtime. He wrapped his hand in the red cloth and dabbed his clothed forefinger in the fudgy white stuff. Then, in a carefully widening spiral, he painted it on the surface of the table, rubbing it wider and wider until, with more applications and new spirals, the whole of the surface had been covered and there was no visible trace of wax to be seen. He went on rubbing, with the heel of the palm, until it was all absorbed by the cherry-wood, even though it was not yet shining. He tidily folded the red cloth and placed it on the sideboard next to the tin of wax, which he sealed. Then he took the blue cloth, and patiently, drifting into a state of mild dreaming concentration, he buffed the surface until it shone. Until he could see his face in it. That was his grandfather's expression.

His grandfather had said this when he was eight years old, years ago. That was when he had last seen him.

At the end, when the table was clean and dry and he could see his face in it, he placed his schoolwork and the laptop in the sideboard drawer reserved for them. He took the cloths and the wax and returned them to the cupboard under the kitchen sink. Then, as today, he started on the next part of his task, of taking the cutlery out, three knives and three forks and three spoons, three water glasses, and the table mats for each place and the bigger mats to place in the middle of the table to put hot dishes on. He was allowed to choose the table mats for each place setting, so long as he did not choose the best ones, and today he lingered pleasurably before deciding. After a minute, he had it down to two: either the honeysuckle, or the rabbit and cabbage ones, and the honeysuckle in the end won.

He clashed around a little in the kitchen, banging knives and forks together as he collected them. It worked. It was a quarter to six. His mother opened the door of the sitting room and came out into the hallway, stretching her shoulders back in that way she had. She had a blue sweater on. She was pretty, William's mother; the blue of this sweater was ugly and dead-looking, but still she was pretty.

You've been busy, she said.

William spread his hands modestly, and carried on with his tasks.

Have you polished the table? she said. I can smell. It's delicious.

Can you say delicious about things you can't eat? William said.

Hmm, his mother said. That was the sound she made, not when she was thinking, but when she wanted people to think that she was thinking. The note she made started high and slid downwards quickly. When she was genuinely thinking, she struck a note with her voice and sustained it. Hmm. I think you're technically correct. But I feel as if I could eat beeswax, it's so good to smell. You're delicious, too. When you were a baby I sometimes wanted to lick you.

Mummy.

Perhaps it's a sort of metaphor. You should ask your father when he asks you about today's new word over dinner.

The sunshine in the park was delicious today, William said.

I think your father would object to that, his mother said.

And it appeared that the door to the study upstairs had been open, his father listening to everything that had been said, observing the life that had been going on in the house, because his father's deep voice now said, Object to what? The words were slow and heavy, as if he had been preparing them for some time.

To the word delicious, wrongly used, his mother said.

And what would the correct word have been, his father's voice came from upstairs, patiently insisting.

Perhaps I should have said delectable, William said.

There was a long silence. His mother looked at him, and he looked at his mother, waiting.

That would have been more appropriate, his father's voice said.

I'm going to cook your dinner now, his mother said. She went into the kitchen, taking the apron from the back of the door, and washed her hands clean – washed them of the burdens of the day, it might have been.

An oneiromantic revelation, I said.

I don't know what those words mean, he said.

Oneiro, to do with dreams, from Greek, I said, and mantic, mancy, something to do with divination, or understanding, I think. Oneiromancy or did I say oneiromantic, the interpretation of dreams, or the meaning of dreams.

Why did you say that, he said.

I had an absolutely extraordinary dream, I said. Sleeping just now on the sofa in the afternoon. It feels so prophetic, no, insightful, no, I think I mean explicatory but I just don't know why. And in a moment I'll forget it. Can I –

Go on, he said.

Mark was there, I said. In some sort of marketplace. He was naked in this crowd and we were there, clothed. And we hailed him and he seemed very proud of something. And then I saw and I said –

What? he said.

No, I said. He explained. All the time people passing by, paying no attention, all this, completely normal, the new ordinary that they were by now quite used to. Mark said that, yes, as we could see, he had had gender reassignment surgery, but though he said that, he was quite the same in all the details. He just had one difference, which was between his legs. And he said very proudly that now he could do what he had always dreamt of doing, and he bent his forehead to the floor and pissed backwards, between his thighs, a big forceful stream.

That is a very odd dream, he said.

And while he was pissing he went on explaining, that now he was retromingent, which in my dream meant he could piss backwards. I don't know, maybe it's also the real word for being able to piss backwards, I'm not sure. The point of the dream was to introduce the word retromingent, I saw that. When the word appeared in the dream I realized that the whole scenario had been presented to me to define the word, like a definition in a dictionary leading up to the word itself.

And how did the word appear in the dream, he said. What was the word?

Retromingent, I said. I was explaining the word to the other people in the dream, like Mark.

Like you're explaining the word to me now, in real life, he said.

Much like that, I said. Words are important and new words are especially important, even if you never use them.

He has a retromingent personality, he said.

I feel a bit odd, I said.

We had not left the house all day. It had rained steadily since I had come back from my parents' house. In the Underground from St Pancras the atmosphere had been thick, a heated and steaming November interior among steaming strangers in their overcoats. I had come into the house, kissed my husband, taken my coat and shoes off and settled on the sofa. I had remained there. The view from the sofa into the street had grown lighter and greyer; darker and blacker; we had opened the curtains and had closed them again. Once a man from the online super-market delivery service had come with crates of food; we had organized the delivery nearly two weeks before in a spirit of whim and sudden urges, and the substance of the delivery came as a series of surprises. Now the kitchen cupboards were full of tinned tropical fruit, bottles of Chinese fish sauces, herbs both dried and fresh, MSG, trotters, flightless birds in tin cans, one lemon.

I felt strange. That is an inadequate way of putting it. Enquiry produces the same response – I don't know. Just strange. And perhaps it is the onset of the strangeness that makes no other answer possible, reduces us through the persistence of illness to the monosyllables we could produce at three years old. I feel strange. What was that strangeness? A veil came between me and the world. At the beginning of the evening, the pair of us sitting on the sofa, the evening news on, the world was quite normal. At eight, as the other evening news we watched was coming to an end, something had come between me and the world. The amplified voices had a sort of echo; the colours were muted and at the same time yellowish.

It's Liam, my husband said, about the cheery weather fore-caster.

I said nothing.

You always say something about Liam, my husband said.

That Liam, I said. He's got a saucy glint in his eye. There's a camerawoman he's keen on.

But my heart was not in it, and my husband asked if I was tired. I agreed that I was: I ached at ankle, knee, elbow, neck, head and shoulders, ached at every bony corner, aching with heat and chills.

I'm just tired, I said. It was getting back from Sheffield this afternoon, it took it out of me.

You came back three days ago, he said.

Well, I'm still tired, I said. I might have an early night.

How could you think you'd come back from Sheffield this afternoon.

I wasn't thinking straight. Early night.

It's eight o'clock.

There's no law against it, I said. I got up. In ten minutes my face was washed; I put on my pyjamas; I went to bed with a copy of *Villette*, a novel I had always loved. Lucy Snowe was in agonies of isolation and boredom; in the town of Villette, she ventured out to a church to confess, just to have someone else to talk to. *The solitude and the stillness of the long dormitory could not be borne any longer; the ghastly white beds were turning into spectres – the coronal of each became a death's head, huge and sun-bleached – dead dreams of an elder world and mightier race lay frozen in their wide gaping eye-holes.* I read the sentence again. The word *coronal* paused me. I had no idea what it meant, and when I read the sentence for a third time I could understand nothing else in it. Sleep was seizing me, like a peeled orange being crushed of juice by a muscular and practised fist, draining me of anything like power. Now it is only eight o'clock, I said, as oblivion and darkness took me down into an unconsciousness more like fainting than sleep. The voices from the other room continued. The day that had passed receded into a gap between hot dreams. Those fevered dreams of mine, after what seemed quite some time, incorporated the words I must have been overhearing, the faint but unarguable tune introducing a comedy of sinister and heated impact. I stood back. I watched. I shivered.

The mother had prepared the meat mixture for the shepherd's pie earlier. She had made an Italian ragù, quickly chopping an onion, a carrot, a stick of celery. In the fifteen minutes after breakfast, when the father had removed himself to his upper study, she had let the *soffritto* soften in oil in a large pan. William was emptying the dishwasher of yesterday's plates, and now loading it with the breakfast things. When it was full, the programme would be run, as they went to bed tonight. She added the meat, stirring it, then a pint of milk and three tins of tomatoes. The wet mixture would sit on the stove, simmering away, for some hours, harmlessly. When she came out from the sitting room for the mid-morning coffee, it was done. She covered it and turned off the gas.

Now all that needed to be done was to boil and mash the potatoes and place the pie in the oven. She liked to cook. When they had first married, she had set about expanding the small repertoire she had acquired as a student, living in that flat in Streatham with the two girls, taking a break from her economics master's thesis with attempts on Italian dishes, learning how risotto was made and what a proper lasagne looked like. And what ragù was. Those investigations expanded in the first year of being married to Femi; sardines married to saffron and sultanas and pasta, chickens boned and stuffed, veal finished with Marsala wine. She had thought it would show love. She liked doing it, too. One day Femi said to her that he didn't know why she put herself to so much trouble. She had taken it down a notch. These days, dinners ran, more or less, according to a schedule two weeks long, with leftovers eaten the next day at lunch.

Some days she thought she might die. That was not an idiom or a turn of phrase. Some days she looked at the dish she was cooking, which was exactly the same as the dish she had permitted herself to cook two Tuesdays ago. She would remem-

tional tying up of shoelaces; the front door was borderline slammed. There was nothing more to do in the kitchen. Dara took her mobile phone from the work surface, and sat at a chair by the table. She dialled; she spoke. She could not be alone with her thoughts.

How we understand the world is the same as how the novel understands and reproduces the world. One of the subjects it, and we, look at is what we cannot see; what we can only see the physical results of; what happens inside a head that is not ours.

The reader should know that the novelist tries to explain what drives a character; what they think and what they believe. And there are ways in which the novelist can do this. There is the same way that we try to understand what a person in real life thinks or believes. That is to present a character's external surface, his or her gestures and expressions and how their speech or silences betray what might be going on inside. But in real life many people are slow to understand those leakages, and may not understand what the novelist understands by a single gesture. If I wrote *The front door closed behind Femi and William. Dara, alone in the kitchen, passed her hand rapidly over her forehead* it might not be agreed by any two readers what that gesture of the hand meant. The novel would have to amplify, *passed her hand rapidly over her forehead in a gesture of relief*, or *irritation*, or *mild despair*. The reader would be guided.

Or the novel can indulge itself in doing what no real person can do: pass without effort into the head of a character, to report the thoughts of the character as articulate, fully formed and in coherent sentences. *Dara thought that though she loved her husband, he had grown tetchy and difficult in the last few weeks under lockdown, and she sometimes wondered whether a serious depression was at the root of his behaviour.* It would be so easy. But all characters have thoughts that are much the same;

they talk differently, but their thoughts are indistinguishable. It feels too easy to leap into a character's head to explain things, and too remote from the real process of thinking, of single words or phrases, of bursts of strongly felt word groupings, of images, tunes, remembered smells and tastes and other word-less things beyond the power of a verbal medium to render. The novel of characters' thoughts has come to seem lazy and childish to me, like an infant granting itself the power of flight or invisibility without any real knowledge of what it will do with it.

Or there is what I think I will do with Dara, an artificial and rigid convention with no real plausibility in life today. There is a class of characters in literature called the *confidante* and I think I will grant Dara one, a character not required to have any life of her own, just a posited existence paying attention to what the heroine tells her about her life and drama, to offer sympathy, to bring objects on command that will advance the plot, to explain matters to the reader or audience. There are maidservants in Shakespeare; there is a couple in a novel by Henry James called *The Golden Bowl* who do nothing but explain the doings of the major characters to each other; there is a novel I love by Tove Jansson, *Moominland in November*, where all the main characters have left, and all that are left are the confidants, trying without success to confide what they have learnt in each other. Yes: let Dara have a confidante. Who she is does not matter; she will receive the inner pain of Dara like a deep, thick-glazed bowl in which biting poisons can be blended with safety. She is on the phone.

I think I might just walk out, Dara said.

Some days, do you have this, Dara said. It's like I've got nothing left.

Of course I know, Dara said. I'm a good mother. I'm not walking out on William, leaving him with Mr That's-known-as-cottage-pie. I can't take him either. Where would I go, Where would I go.

Well, that's good of you but we're talking for ever, not a week or two, Dara said. And then would he manage – Femi?

It's not normal, him being like this, Dara said. He has his ritual. He gets up at seven sharp. He goes for his run, an hour exactly. I know what that means. He runs to Battersea Park and he does three circuits of the whole park. He comes back and he showers and we have breakfast at twenty minutes past eight. Yesterday's leftovers at one o'clock; another run just before dinner. The rest of the time, the whole of the rest of the time, he is in his room, working. I see something wrong when I look at him, something wrong in his eyes.

One day I am going to kill him if things don't change, Dara said. I mustn't keep you. Listen to me going on like this. It's not that bad, not really.

Dara ended the call. She put the phone into her pocket. The kitchen was tidy, the pie heating in the oven, the pan of water on the stove waiting for the heat to be turned on and the frozen peas poured in. The dining room was tidy, the table shining and smelling of wax polish, neatly set for dinner by William, who had put all his books and papers away. She went to the sitting room and did the same thing at the little desk in the corner, tidying her papers and closing the file she'd been working on, a curriculum thing. When the papers were in two squared-off piles she went around the room, shaking each cushion, placing the two remote controls square on the table by Femi's place on the sofa, picking up a stray glass she had somehow overlooked the day before. One book was missing from the case where the sets of books were kept in a neat array, the white-and-black-edged spines of English classics. William must have taken it to read, but he would return it to its place. She could turn on the television to watch the news, but she thought she would not. There was nothing much to do but wait for the pie to finish cooking and for her husband and son to return. The word of the day: nothing much.

William and his father left the house. The boy benefited from these outings with his father. He was bookish, shy, withdrawn. That was not the recipe for social popularity and likeability, things of undoubted significance in life. *Mens sana in corpore sano* had been translated for Femi in the assembly hall of his school in Streatham, twenty-five years ago. A healthy mind in a healthy body. There had been a line of incredulous white liberal adults behind the strict headmistress who, like Femi, knew the value of education. She had benefited from it. One of the first Black headmistresses in the country, he believed, even in the 1990s. In his mind the Latin tag meant outdoors. When the boy was a little older he would take him out running or similar exercise. Now his indoors life – the screens every child now lived by as well as the books that were more unusual and probably marked William out as distinct from his peers – could be extended and diverted by these small outings.

The evening was dry and dark and cold. The street was silent. They had lived here for ten years now, moving for an extra bedroom William could grow up in and another bedroom for the second child that had never come. They had stretched themselves then in financial terms. Six months ago he had thought that they could stretch themselves again. But now there seemed no point. They would stay here until things came to an end.

Look at that, Femi said to his son. He already felt a little splendid; the dry martini in a tumbler downstairs in the kitchen and the one or two before it, upstairs in the study in his water glass, the bottle he kept on the bookshelf. It was a series of dry martinis with no ice and no vermouth, which had no need of a martini glass. And now he felt up to the world in dry darkness.

It's a cherry tree, I think, William said, after a moment. Femi had been indicating what was behind the tree, a bright yellow Mini Cooper he had never seen before in the street. He let it go.

How do you know, Femi said.

I compared it with *The Observer's Book of Trees*, William said. It's the bark, look, the way it sort of peels back in that shiny way. People who like trees go mad for that. It must be a bit untidy in a garden.

Does it … Femi said. He struggled for a moment to say what he wanted to say. Does it … peel away? Fall down?

William did not answer, perhaps because the words his father had used for the process were not the correct ones an expert would use. To split; to shed; to debride; to peel.

Did you have a new word today? Femi said.

Recalcitrant, William said. He gave both Cs a hard pronunciation; then he mulled and said it again, and again. The third time he said it he was satisfied it was correct. Recalcitrant. Recalcitrant. It means unwilling, if you won't do as you're told. You children are being very recalcitrant today.

Did your teacher use it?

No, William said. She'd never use a word like recalcitrant. I don't think she knows words like that.

I'm sure she knows, Femi said. She is a teacher, after all. You might never have heard her use the word, but she will definitely know it. Respect.

I don't think so, William said. When she asked everyone in the class what they were reading last week and I said *Jorrocks' Jaunts and Jollities* she'd never heard of it. Then she said she didn't like books from the old-fashioned times, that's what she said. And then when she heard it was about hunting she pulled a face and asked the next kid whether they would ever read a book like that.

What did they say?

I don't care what they said, William said. It's a matter of indifference to me whether those people read at all, so long as they don't stop me reading what I want.

And that is an example of recalcitrancy, Femi said.

So it is, William said.

But you should never criticize a teacher, Femi said. That is very disrespectful.

Without the slightest warning, he cuffed William about the head; it was not a joking cuff. He hit him, and hard.

I woke in the night and was shivering. I was woken in the night by my shivering. Shivering did not cover it. It was electric, convulsive, eruptive, shaking the bed and drumming on the floor. My muscles were in spasm, and the pillow and sheets I lay on were wet as if I had slept through a rainstorm.

My husband was there and then he was not there. I remembered he had not been in the bed when I fell asleep, too early. On the bedside table the clock said 4:23 but that made no sense, that was teatime in the afternoon, the clock was wrong and broken, and as I thought that the clock changed and it was 4:24 and I remembered this time happened as well in the night when usually I was asleep. My husband was back and the light was on. The light had been on when I had woken up. He must have put it on unless he was just coming to bed. He put his hand on my forehead and said, with a kind of wonder, Shivering. He had in his hand a small white thermometer. He waited. In a while the most violent shivering abated; I no longer felt as if I were carrying out some strenuous exercise. He pressed a button, extracting a single beeping noise, and put it underneath my tongue. I did not speak; the judders and twitches and spasms continued in waves.

I had a terror of violent shivering, though I had been told that I was very good at it. Once a friend at university, whom I shared a decrepit house with, itself shuddering with ill-fitting windows, came down to breakfast in January to find me hunched over my cornflakes, my jaw crashing violently with the sheer cold of an English terraced house with no working heating or insulation. I knew you liked novels, the friend said with some disgust. I never thought you'd take it as far as getting your teeth to chatter. I asked what he meant; it turned out that he believed that the chattering of teeth was a literary invention, a trope that bore no relation to anything the body might really do. There were such inventions, I know, but the chattering of my teeth was quite genuine. And there were, too, the episodes of shivering that come with significant infections I had known in hospital beds; the peritonitis that had followed an appendix removal when I was fourteen had culminated in two days of shattering spasms. I remembered my upper arms tight against my sides, my shoulders juddering and grinding, the look of sheer terror on my mother's face as she was bundled off. It had happened, again, in hospital the year before, as an infection took its course, the bed vibrating with the force of my trembling, two friends visiting politely looking away with concern and a disconcerting respect for my illness's waywardness. Now I had a fever, in my own bed at home, and the shivering was as bad as it had ever been.

It's going to be me next, I expect, my husband said. He looked at the temperature reading. Thirty-nine. That's not ideal. How do you feel?

Not, I started to say, but my jaw would not let me get anything much out.

I'll get a test, my husband said. What he said did not seem to make any sense. Who would test my husband and what were they going to test him on. A glass of water was there and a pill and then nothing again and darkness. Somewhere in the hour since I had woken up shivering I had sat in the bedroom armchair while he took off the wet sheets, the wet pillowcases, the wet cover of the duvet, and put new clean dry ones on, the red one I liked. I changed my pyjamas. We turned out the light. In a few minutes I was shivering again. The pyjamas I wore and the sheets underneath me began to feel warm and damp, and then wet with sweat.

A virus may be transmitted directly, or in this case indirectly, through fomite transmission or contact with contaminated surfaces, such as a metal pole in a train carriage. Once the droplet particles from an infectious person are transferred to a surface, another person can place his hand on that surface, pick up the infection within the deposited droplet particles. When his hand next comes into contact with his eyes, nose or mouth, or when he inhales aerosol particles from an infected person in the air, the virus may be transmitted.

The virus that is under question is a variety of coronavirus, named after a distinctive shape of the transmitting molecule. This variety is known as SARS-CoV, named after its ability to cause severe acute respiratory syndrome. Acute does not indicate severity, but the speed of onset; severe indicates severity. The virus enters the host cell by binding to angiotensin-converting enzymes. It will then infect the epithelial cells within the lungs.

The first symptoms for the patient are a high temperature, often accompanied by constant coughing. A loss of smell and taste may occur. Tiredness and difficulty breathing are common indicators. In some patients, the difficulty breathing may lead to oxygen shortage, which may in turn lead to confusion and delirium. In time the patient may have difficulty breathing and artificial aids may be necessary. It has been noted that after the first week of symptoms, patients either start to recover, or experience a worsening of the condition, which may lead to death. Comorbidities, such as obesity, hypertension, heart disease, often identify patients more likely to die. When death occurs, it is normally due to septic shock and the failure of multiple organs, caused by an infection in the lungs. A smaller number are killed by respiratory failure caused by diffuse alveolar damage.

Deaths worldwide due to the Covid virus currently stand at 5.33 million. Those over 55 provide the greater number of deaths in all territories, from slightly over 55 per cent in Bangladesh to nearly 100 per cent in Western Europe. Vaccines began to be applied to the general public in some countries in the spring of 2021. At the end of November 2020 I was fifty-five years old, and I contracted the SARS-CoV1 virus, transmitting it unknowingly and immediately to my husband, who was fifty years and three months old.

I wonder what it is goes on in his skull, Dara said. She said it out loud, in the empty house. But she felt she knew the answer. When he spoke to her about what had happened in his day, upstairs in the study, it was often about moments when he had bested or humiliated a colleague. She rarely believed these stories; they were so invariant in their conclusions, and co-opted an invisible horde into support for the thing he'd said, the action he'd taken.

When he was alone and imagining things, she felt, he would be constructing scenes to come. The woman in the shop said to me – so I said – and she said – and I pointed out – and she said – and I put the basket down on the counter and told her that if she wanted to be like that, I'd be doing my shopping elsewhere. None of any of this would have happened. Her husband spent his imaginative energies thinking up offensive or confrontational things people might say to him in order to allow himself a triumph.

One of those triumphs would be over her. The conversations between them, late at night as they prepared themselves for bed, had hardened into a regularized, even an ideal, form. She knew exactly how they ran by now, in general. She heard them as clearly as if they were happening just at this moment, above her head.

I wish you wouldn't speak to me like that.

When the boy's there, you mean.

Not just that. I wish you wouldn't speak to me like that at all.

Men don't speak to their wives like that, you mean. Or you don't think they should.

I don't know whether they do or not, but I wish you wouldn't. And, yes, I don't think you should do it in front of William.

You think I set him a bad example.

I think it frightens him.

That's rubbish.

Why is it rubbish?

If you don't want him to be frightened, you shouldn't have done what you did.

I thought we were finished with that.

With Mr Rupert Fitchwell? With your Rupert? I don't know why you should think we'll ever be finished with that.

You can't help yourself.

I can't be expected to forget about it, to forget what you did to our marriage.

No.

And again Mr Rupert Fitchwell was in the house they shared, the bedroom they had shared for fifteen years. The house rang with his sonorous clang, the contemptuous spit of his name, and the bedroom vibrated with his presence, like the inside of a great bell. It would not even be true to say that she succeeded in putting him from her mind. He was never in her mind. The past entered into the space, into the present moment not just of experience but of telling, too. He had put it there by his pained and inevitable use of the name he hated, the name he had installed in his head.

And the teller brings the past into the room of the present. The past is always with us, and the novelist knows that. The present moment, which we feel contains the past, is brought alongside that past on precisely the same terms by the act of telling in prose. We always find it easy to say something not just about the present moment we happen to be observing but, on the same level as the present event, a sentence about the past that has shaped the present, a sentence like *Many years before, Daphne had seduced Caroline's father; even now, Caroline found it hard to talk openly about anything to Daphne* is dropped in, and we return in a moment to the conversation between two women. The novel tells about the present, but it knows how to bring the past into the room, and it does so without fuss or artifice, as if the past is always there in the air. The past is always there, in the air we breathe. And so –

Rupert Fitchwell was a parent. He was familiar to Dara by reputation, and to her school by experience. He had sent five children to the school, one after another, starting twelve years before – the first, Sonia Fitchwell, had gone to Durham University to read French, was now working for an estate agent in Guildford. The children were cowed, conventional, popular because of their good looks – they were mixed race, their eyes glacial and cryptic, their faces stretched tight over what had been referred to as *good bone structure*. The mother, presumably Black, was not seen; Rupert Fitchwell, a white solicitor, was known to almost everybody. His intrusions and his sayings were passed around the staff room. The first thing Dara heard about him was that he had said he wasn't going to pay for educating five children – three and it might be a possibility, but five and they'd have to take their chances.

Take their chances meant *be educated by the professional that I happen to be speaking to.* It irritated the member of staff, and she shared it widely. Rupert Fitchwell always lobbied hard on behalf of his children, even the middle one, Linus, who had to have everything explained to him twice, once after the lesson had finished, with little ultimate effect. Rupert Fitchwell always made a point, when meeting a new member of staff, of saying that his marriage was successful because of their cultural differences, and that he had always found Black women attractive; one thing impossible to debate or argue over, there it was. The Black woman teacher he would be talking to would say nothing, and let the observation lie where it was, satisfied with itself.

Dara had never met him. A message came through that Mr Rupert Fitchwell was concerned about his youngest child, Sylvia, and would welcome a meeting with the head teacher. A message was passed back that he should arrange a meeting with Sylvia's form teacher; Sue Spark was generous with her own time, and would certainly not object to meeting him for half an hour after school one day, or speaking to him on the phone at his convenience. That would not do: he had concerns about Mrs Spark, too. After some time a meeting was arranged. Dara apologized to Sue Spark and made it plain that no criticism of her would be taken seriously. She knew Rupert Fitchwell or, if not him, then she knew the type. A meeting was arranged between the head teacher, Dara, and Rupert Fitchwell at 5 p.m. on Friday, 24 January 2020, to take place in the head teacher's office at the school.

In the night I felt bad. Sweat ran from me. It was three. Then it was five. I got up and I was hot and the bed was wet, like hot rain had soaked it. There was the thing that went under the tongue and the thing that went on your hand. I used them.

Are you ill.

Yes. I feel bad. Worse than.

Worse than.

Yes. Worse than last night.

This is the third day.

I think it's the fourth.

Let's change the bed.

I was shaking and shaking. He was shaking and shaking too. We took the sheet off and put a new one on, a dry one, and then the same for the quilt. I sat with the thing under my tongue. I took it out. It showed a number and the number showed I was ill. I changed my clothes and we got back into bed. It was six and it was dark and I slept.

The room had some light in it. The things were open, the curtains. How were they open. I could smell my wet body. I was ill. I got out of bed and then it was too much. I sat in the chair by the bed. The room was far from me, it was dead, it was wrapped like in wool. The walls were red as before and on them were small pictures and big pictures, faces and shapes and people who were dead, and a stretch of land and a road in snow. There were doors, and clothes hung behind the closed doors. It was my house and it was strange. There was a noise in my ear like a long thud that did not stop.

I feel bad.

I feel bad too.

I need a bath.

I got up from the chair and I went to the room with the bath in it. At some point I went on my knees and stayed there for a while. I ran the bath and got in it. When I got in it was hot and when I got out it was cold. My arm shook and my teeth banged, like it was cold, but I was ill and that was all.

He was where he had been, in the bed.

Have you, have you, he said.

I knew what he meant. Yes. It's high.

How high.

It's. It's thirty-nine and a half. I think.

Is that high.

That's high. What's yours.

I don't know. Give it to me.

Time went by and he lay in the bed with his head flat and the white thing in his mouth. There was nothing in my head but I could wait. The white thing made a sound, the thermometer.

The thermometer, I said.

Look.

That's high as well.

Have you done the other thing, the breath thing, oxygen.

I went to the drawer and took the other thing out, the oximeter, and it went on my hand, my finger.

It's low.

How low.

I showed him. It said ninety-three.

Let me try, he said. Then later he said, Mine's all right.

We sat there for a time. I cried and then I stopped. I got up and I opened the doors where the clothes were. I took off my night clothes and I put on my day clothes. I put on blue jeans and red socks and a shirt with vines on it, a pattern, a design. I looked at him when I was dressed. His eyes were closed and he lay in bed. His face was pink as well as brown.

Your face is pink as well as brown, I said.

I feel bad, he said.

I had to get up. If I did not get up I would be more than ill. He could not get up and it was best for him not to get up. I went into another room, where the food was, the kitchen. The fridge had food in it and the doors hid more food, the cupboards, but I could not eat. It must have been two days since I ate. I was there for a while and I did not think and I did not know anything.

The street was on the other side of the door and the world was there and I was in here and so was he and we were ill, wrapped in wool, our mouths open and our arms limp with ache. I took a pill. Then I drank a glass. Time went by and it was ten. I took a glass and a pill to where he was, in bed, in a state of sleep. I woke him and gave them to him. He told me that he had an ache and I said I had an ache too. I picked up a book and I went to another room and I lay down. The book was in my hand. I read some words and they made no sense.

The empty lodging-house rustled with sea noises, as though years of echoes of waves and sea-sucking shingle lived in its chimneys, its half-open cupboards.

House rustled with sea
Sucking shingle lived
Waves and sea sucking
Years of echoes

I read it and it made no sense. I had read this book and it had made sense but now it made no sense and it was the fault of the book. I shut the book and it was called *The Death of the Heart* and I read those five words and they made some sense but not much.

I had read books but now I could not read books and it was gone.

There were two black things on the arm of the chair and I pressed one and then pressed both of them and the thing came on, the screen, television, and noise started. The black things were called remote controls. In front of me there was a face in a room and it spoke and it moved and I watched it. Time went by.

The head teacher's office had been Dara's for three years now, but she had made few changes in it. There was a bookcase in it, which held a few reference books, very few of which needed to be consulted when their information was available on the internet – an atlas, a *Chambers Dictionary*, a *Whitaker's Almanac* for 2004, a volume of *Who's Who* even older. She had thrown away the volumes of the London phone directory and a *Yellow Pages*, not having consulted them for many years, and had added very few books to the shelves – a French dictionary and her grandfather's magnum opus on Nigerian taxation law, probably useless but impressive for show. In recent weeks, she had ordered and placed on the shelves a copy of a reference work about trees in Britain; she had intended to master it in her spare time to keep up with William's interest. But there was no time and no keeping up with an eleven-year-old boy's burning interest – a blazing front of all-consuming flame.

The pleasant green and brown curtains had been inherited from Kate Lingard, the previous head, who had retired after twelve years in the post. There was a desk for working, three armchairs around a coffee-table, all in the same matching stuff. The yellowish-brown furniture, looking as if it would be sticky to the touch, had been the school's property for decades longer, as had the grey carpet and the large vase with a pattern of interlocking fish. Dara kept that empty, not being a fan of cut flowers in an office. Kate Lingard had had a Persian carpet underneath the coffee-table, an indicator of status and cool respectability, but she had taken that with her. Taken, too, a squat pottery bowl with an ultramarine glaze from the coffee-table; an object, Kate Lingard would tell visitors, that had been made for her by a student she'd been advised to give up on, but hadn't. There you are, you see. In Kate Lingard's day, the ultramarine bowl had been a useful parable of labour rewarded. Dara was surprised that she'd taken it with her. Nobody so far had given her a bowl to reward her trust and goodwill, and the coffee-table stood empty. The only things she had brought with her into the office were a photograph of her, William and Femi on holiday in Italy, five years ago when William was quite small, and a Nespresso machine. Kate Lingard had got Carol in the outer office to make her coffees; Dara didn't feel she could do that, and saw no need now that coffee from capsules was so excellent. She did her job. Her office was at the corner of the building, with views over the city on the east side of the building, over the playground and down to the woods on the north.

Rupert Fitchwell was on time. Carol showed him in, saying as she did so that if there was no more work for her, she'd be leaving now.

Poets' Day, Rupert Fitchwell said. That's what we used to call Friday in the old days.

Why poets? Dara said.

Piss off early, tomorrow's Saturday, Rupert Fitchwell said, and sat down in one of the armchairs, dropping his leather satchel on the floor. He was a tall man; with dark eyebrows, bulging thyroidal blue eyes and a mouth too broad for his face, he would have been an effective stage actor, his performed emotions visible from far off.

You're not leaving early, Dara said to Carol, ignoring this. It's after five. Thank you so much for everything.

Carol went, shutting the door with unnecessary calm and carefulness.

They told me about you, Rupert Fitchwell said.

Just a second, Dara said. She went to her desk; while still standing up she wrote a couple of final sentences to the email she had been typing; she pressed send. Now. It's Mr Fitchwell, isn't it? I don't think we've met before.

I would certainly remember.

You say that you're concerned about Sylvia.

Yes, Rupert Fitchwell said. He fell into silence, rather openly inspecting Dara. She had seen this before: people who had not been told enough about the head teacher they were there to meet, and who had perhaps wanted to ask if they could see her credentials before continuing. There was something in that here, but also something of the sizing up, the assessor, the contestant in a guess-your-weight game.

Perhaps you could say what the areas of concern are.

I've got five children, Rupert Fitchwell said. May I say that we have always been very pleased with the school?

Thank you.

Sylvia's a very sensitive child. She doesn't need to be ridiculed. He gazed without blinking; a liar.

I think we can agree that children shouldn't be ridiculed, but could you explain?

You wanted me to meet with her form mistress.

Form teacher. Sue Spark, yes.

But the trouble is that Ms Sparks seems to hate Sylvia for no reason and ridicules her in front of the whole class.

In what way?

She once asked Sylvia if she was a lesbian, because she looked like one when she came with her hair tied back. I think it all began when Sylvia borrowed a marker pen from the whiteboard without asking and forgot to give it back.

Let's not get into the marker pen, Dara said, writing down SS. Said looks like lesbian. Are you sure that's what Mrs Spark said?

Quite sure, Rupert Fitchwell said. And another time. She told Sylvia that she was glad she wasn't a half-caste like her. I was really very surprised that anyone in two thousand and twenty was still talking in such a way.

Dara noted irrelevantly that Rupert Fitchwell was still saying two thousand when everyone had changed to twenty twenty; it had been a bugbear of Femi's for as long as she had known him, that people should have said twenty hundred. Her husband's voice popped into her head, as it did. What was popping into Rupert Fitchwell's head? Some triumph.

I am very surprised, too. May I ask why you are certain that an experienced teacher like Mrs Spark said such things? I've worked closely with her for some years. I would have said she was among the fairest and most patient of my teachers. The most fair.

Not in Sylvia's experience.

Disconcertingly, Rupert Fitchwell grinned; his wide mouth split his face. There was a dusting of hair on his chin, gingerish as many Englishmen were. She supposed he must have been good-looking before he acquired the basset-hound expression.

You've got to agree, Rupert Fitchwell said, that your Miss Sparks is a copper-bottomed cunt in the old style.

Mr Fitchwell.

Should I apologize?

Have you heard this from anyone but Sylvia?

Do you think she would make something like this up?

The answer to that was yes, of course, but Dara went on. What Rupert Fitchwell's reason was for coming here with some child's fantasy about the abuse they had suffered, she could not say. In the end they agreed that Rupert Fitchwell would ask his daughter in a more sceptical way. Interrogative, like a barrister, Dara had said. In the end, Rupert Fitchwell got up and shook her hand. It was only a quarter past five; she would stay a little longer. At the door he paused.

There's something else you might like to know, he said. My wife came back to me. After leaving the marital home. I thought we were heading for divorce but apparently not.

That must be a relief. I'm pleased to hear it.

It has been difficult but I'm sure the effect on the children won't be lasting.

I'm sure you will be there for them.

Nobody from the school got in touch, you know. To ask if things were all right.

I'm sorry, Mr Fitchwell, Dara said formally. I have to confess, this is the first I've heard of your wife having left you, let alone coming back. If we seemed heartless, that was probably because we just didn't know.

We, Rupert Fitchwell said. That confirmed something for Rupert Fitchwell. He murmured something that might have been Good, good, and left.

That night she did not mention Rupert Fitchwell. Why should she? It was completely trivial; it had no interest for anyone else. Instead, the conversation had been about shoes.

You don't have anything to do tomorrow, do you? William. William. Don't read at the dining table. I was asking if you had anything to do tomorrow. I'm going to take you to buy some new trainers. Would you like that?

I don't really need new trainers, William said. The ones I've got, the black ones with the white bits on, we got them after my birthday.

I thought we'd go up to the West End, Dara said. For once. Don't you want some cooler trainers than those?

Don't make him dissatisfied with what he's got, Femi said.

I like those trainers, William said. They're really comfy.

I got them from Marks and Spencer, Dara said. In an emergency. Mainly because I knew if they weren't right you could take them back.

But they're fine, William said, puzzled. You didn't have to take them back.

William, don't tell me that the cool kids in your class think they're cool.

I don't care what that lot think about anything. They're only cool because they can't do anything – they can't do quadratic equations even – and they sit at the back pretending they're too street to be bothered with anything hard. They're idiots.

Have the idiots made any observations about your trainers, Femi said, with the tremor of a chuckle.

I don't think so, William said. I wouldn't pay any attention if they did.

You're a strange boy, Dara had said. He had these fits of stubbornness; she never knew when they would come up. She knew Femi would only say that he should be proud of who he was, and later that night, when William had gone to bed, Femi embarked on one of his reasonable explanations. It was more rambling and repetitious than it might once have been, because by nine o'clock Femi was drunk on a sequence of his gin cocktails, but it was still reasonable. She wanted her son to be one of the cool kids and admired for the trainers he had on. William had made a very good point in saying that the supposedly cool kids were frightened of attempting anything they might fall short on. Those children, therefore, could only be admired for their trainers, which, after all, anybody could buy.

Was she following him?

Yes, she was. But my God, those trainers, she didn't add.

He switched on the bedside radio. The shipping forecast was in progress, the names always familiar and meaningless to her, like the formal statements of love: German Bight; Dogger. They were there to cover any sentence the boy might hear pass between them.

Perhaps if it was so important to her that her son be cool and wear the right clothes, she might have taken this into consideration when she decided to get married. Had it not occurred to her that no son of Femi would inherit any degree of coolness from his father? Hard work, yes. A sense of justice, yes. (Femi ran through his own virtues for two or three minutes.) Those in his view were things worth inheriting. Did she agree? He was glad they were on the same page in this regard. It made him wonder. Femi sat with his hands clasped in front of him. He had not changed on returning from the office as he once had, and he was wearing a blue striped shirt with a white collar, open to the top of one of his string-work vests, and a pair of charcoal grey suit trousers, his feet in grey ribbed socks. She didn't suppose he had worn an item of sportswear when not exercising in his life, or a single piece of clothing with any form of writing on it. It made him wonder.

What did it make him wonder.

It made him wonder why she'd married him in the first place.

Okay, well.

If you had wanted a father of a cool son rather than –

He waved his hand dismissively, in the direction of upstairs.

– maybe you should have married somebody else. A street wastrel in the right trainers. Perhaps you shouldn't have chosen to marry me. My trainers are for running.

I married the man my grandfather chose for me, Dara said. I'm going to bed. I can't be doing with this.

That was Friday and on Saturday morning the letter arrived from Rupert Fitchwell. He had discovered that his wretched daughter had told him a pack of lies. He was so sorry. Could he perhaps take her out to dinner to make amends? They had so much in common, he was sure.

The envelope only bore the words By Hand. (He knew where she lived.) Femi had opened it and read it. He was waiting for her when she came back from the supermarket with William.

There was a smell in the house.

I could smell just one thing.

I was dressed and in the room with the things in it. I must have got up. I lay on the chair, the long chair, the sofa. On the screen men talked. I watched them move. It was light out there.

Then I looked again and it was dark and there was a smell in the house. I called out but my voice was weak. My arms had an ache and my legs had an ache. I felt ill and I knew what it was. I did not know what the day was. There was a noise from the room with the bed in it. It was a voice. It sounded ill too. I stayed where I was.

There was a smell in the house. It smelt like the worst thing for me. The worst thing for me was what the thing, the thing in the place, the kitchen, the stove in the kitchen, what they smell like when they aren't clean. That smell I knew and I hated. The word musty came to my mind. I should clean the stove. It smelt so bad. But then it was true that I had cleaned it, not too long back. I did not like the smell of an old stove so I cleaned it all the time. I did not know where the smell was, then.

There was a sound at the door.

It was the bell. I stood up. It was hard. I walked to the door. That was hard too. My friend Mark stood out there, ten feet off. He smiled.

How are you feeling, he said.

Not great. What's this?

At my feet were six bags from Waitrose.

I thought you would probably need some shopping done.

Oh, darling, I said.

There's nothing that'll need parboiling or flambéing or even peeling, he said. It's just ready meals. And some little treats, a box of éclairs.

You're so sweet.

Don't stand out here, he said. How bad do you feel?

How bad do I look?

Awful. How's your man?

Hasn't got out of bed for a week, I said.

But I did not know. It might have been a week or it might have been two.

How can I pay you back, I said.

Sort it out later, he said. There's a bottle of champagne in there too for when you start to feel on the mend.

I brought the bags in – Mark could not come near. Then I blew a kiss. He went. I shut the door. Out there was the man who lived on the far side of the street. He had seen and heard it all. His name was Neil. I took the bags into the house, and the stuff in the bags went into the fridge or the other place, the thing with doors. Then I went to the room, I lay down, I slept. There was a voice from the screen that went on for a bit and then stopped. When I woke up I could smell the same thing. It had grown and was all round me, like a cloud I could not see. The death of burnt old food in a stove that had not been cleaned.

We live in the world, and to establish how people are, and how they react, I had long ago come to the conclusion that the world must impinge on them. It troubled me in a novel when everything operated under the control of psychologies, and the psychologies never seemed real to me if they could manipulate the resistant world without limit. When I wrote a novel, I often liked to write a draft episode I could leave out later in which a gun was fired outside the house, a gun fired by no one of the slightest importance. Once that had happened and I had seen my characters react to it, I would start to understand them. The world, I think, is a world of things, and the novelists I liked best knew this, and listed their resistant selves, insisting on what they wanted in a world of psychology. The novel I read today, an old favourite, knew this.

Several disordered tables showed that people had already lunched, and left; but in the corner was a table for two, freshly laid in the best manner of such restaurants; that is to say, with a red-and-white checked cloth, and two other red-and-white cloths, almost as large as the tablecloth, folded as serviettes and arranged flat on two thick plates between solid steel cutlery; a salt-cellar, out of which one ground rock-salt by turning a handle, a pepper-castor, two knife-rests, and two common tumblers. The phenomena which differentiated the table from the ordinary table were a champagne bottle and a couple of champagne glasses.

I felt a kind of ecstasy at these sixteen or twenty named objects. They were created to someone's will and devised to draw in another person's desires, and never existed apart from the prose of this novelist. There was no real world of objects, and the illusion of that real world had been created nonetheless. They had wills of their own, and existed apart from the readers' established worlds, the characters', apparently the author's. I had never heard the phrase *pepper-castor*; that made me feel not that the thing it evoked was unreal, but that it had a kind of solidity of existence that was larger than my own range of reference. It must be true; it must have its own ideas of what would happen. Things – mute, resistant things – are important. They set things in motion that we would not initiate, left to ourselves.

In the house, things – familiar, unremarkable things for the most part – had started to appear in wrong and disorderly places, and to stay there. They spoke to her of a mood of urgent neglect, as if they had been cast off just where they were, with irritation and necessity, and left there. One of Femi's socks, cast off on the landing and lying there like a black query on the red carpet; a hardback book with a yellow broken spine abandoned outside on the garden table, open and face down, the memoirs of a Nigerian politician, his sombre face on the cover – that had been a present never intended to be read; foodstuffs started and forgotten about, curved bows of pizza crust, squashed ends of cake like run-over vermin, bright constellations of broken crisps, all this abandoned food on the floor, under chairs. She had mentioned only the food, which could attract vermin. The rest she dealt with.

Now it was a mug on the uppermost shelf of the bookcase in the sitting room. She knew that mug, squat and wide, holding a good pint of coffee. It bore a pattern of abstract diagonal stripes, turquoise and white, dotted with irregular brown dots. It was one of those kitchen objects nobody could remember acquiring, when or why. She worked backwards from the way it had been abandoned. It had been forgotten there; something had distracted him; he had left it where it was; he had been looking at a book on the top shelf, where the never-read and stately volumes lived; he had had to get a chair to stand on to reach that far. She reconstructed the story the right way round. He had come into the room to fetch a book down, had stood on a chair, had placed his mug on the shelf, had taken down the book, forgetting the mug – it made very little sense. The alternative came too quickly to her mind. So much of what he did these days she could construe only as deliberate malice against her, to see how she would deal with something that made no sense.

She pulled the wooden armchair over, and clambered onto it. Even so she had to stretch to reach the mug. It was the wrong weight, not an empty mug, and it unbalanced as she tried to hold it. It must have been nearly full; a splash of cold sour coffee went down her front. She held herself still, her wrist and forearm soaked, her blue sweater drenched. She had the mug; she got down off the chair. At least the carpet and furniture had been spared. The sweater could be soaked and cleaned. Nothing too bad had happened. He had left a full mug of coffee on the top shelf of the bookcase. That was all. By the time Femi and William returned everything would be quite normal.

She disposed of the mug, and went upstairs into their bedroom. An intention had been forming, one she could not quite account for, but she fulfilled it. She closed the curtains and undressed, placing the blue sweater in the laundry basket. It was an awful sweater. It was not even from a clothes shop, but from the large supermarket they always went to. She didn't know why she had bought it – need, almost certainly. She hadn't tried it on and it didn't fit properly. She would put it in the laundry basket and now she would do what she ought to do, put on some clothes she actually liked.

It was a Tuesday night, and the dress she took out of the wardrobe, without hesitation, was not exactly a party dress, but certainly a dress she would have put on if there was a question of meeting other people. It was three or four years old. Dresses like that had been so much the thing, that London summer – floor length, loose, thin as muslin, large swoops of colour, of mustard and purple, of green and orange. Wow, look at you, a friend had said the first time she had worn it out. Is it wearing me, she'd said, remembering that people weren't supposed to notice your clothes, just how well they made you look. You look – wow, you look great, the friend had said.

Is it new, Femi had said. I don't remember it.

Now she stepped into it and it was too much for a Tuesday night, a night with nothing to recommend it, but she felt like it. All nights were the same now; and they were clothes. They might as well be worn. Putting this dress on was a shock of the not-enough. Other clothes she'd felt good in were tight and hard-shaped, the surprisingly heavy yellow cocktail dress, boned and lined and following her pre-William shape that had taken her through their engagement and that first year, or the purple tweed suit with the frayed lapels that had, she explained a dozen times, got her the job of her dreams. This dress was different and at first felt like it hadn't enough grip around her, a loose floating in air. Then it was okay and she liked the way it felt when she walked in it.

Was it a mummy dress? She walked downstairs in it, letting it billow, barefoot. She knew you didn't dress for other people's approval; you dressed for yourself. These days there was only yourself, in any case, and those two others. Femi had never commented; William loved what she wore, and often said, quite out of the blue, You look really pretty in that dress, Mummy. But she dressed for herself and to please herself. She told herself that. The house smelt reassuringly of shepherd's pie; everything was clean; the work for the day was done; her husband and son would return soon; she had made an effort and must be looking pretty good. Tomorrow she would get that blue sweater out of the laundry basket and throw it away. There was the key in the door.

That's your India dress, William said.

Nice walk? she said. He ran to her, the boy; he embraced her, burying his face in her front. She detached him, and gave him a kiss, wondering.

I hate those people, Femi said. I hate them. The world would be a better place without them. I can tell you that for a fact.

Dinner's going to be fifteen minutes, she said. She went into the kitchen. She looked about her. There was nothing to be done. My name is Dara, she said silently. My name is Dara. My name is Dara.

Why does he call it your India dress, Femi said later. He was in the armchair in the bedroom, undressing slowly. He did not look at her. He sat there pulling his socks off with impatient incompetence, as if he had never done this before. He had not looked at her the whole evening.

I don't know, Dara said. He thinks it looks Indian, I suppose. I don't know that it really does.

Rich imagination, Femi said. Not enough effort to make sure he's on top of the facts.

Honestly, I don't know, Dara said.

I suppose you think, Femi said.

You suppose I think what, Dara said quietly and very quickly.

If you did me the courtesy to listen, Femi said, you would find out.

I'm sick of this, Dara said.

Did you think Mr Rupert Fitchwell was at all likely to drop round this evening? Femi said.

Why? Dara said. Did you?

That's a very beautiful and expensive dress you've put on, Femi said. Were you making all that effort just for me?

For my husband, Dara said.

On the television tonight, Femi said. On the television tonight there was a documentary about the Second World War. It was after poor old William went to bed. Didn't want to hear any more of what his daddy had to say.

And who could blame him.

That's as may be. The documentary. Do you know who Admiral Kimmel was? No? American. An admiral. I was struck by his first name. I don't think I ever knew what his first name was. Do you know what his first name was?

Femi tried to stand up, but his ankles were still trapped in his puddled trousers, and he stumbled, falling onto the bed. He continued, supine, working his trousers off with his feet.

His first name was actually Husband. Husband Kimmel. That's interesting, don't you think? I don't know that I've ever heard of a man who was called Husband before. Or a woman, of course.

No.

After the documentary I sat there thinking.

Femi levered himself up; his eyes were bloodshot; he looked straight past Dara at the wall where the snowy landscape hung.

How, Femi said, did they come to that? How would you look at a small baby and think that the name for the baby was going to be Husband. I mean I'm all in favour of not calling babies Buddy and Timmy and Petal and names only a baby could have, but Husband …

It must have been a family name, Dara said.

And when he met his wife, Femi said, did he say to her, Call me Husband, and did she call him Husband? And at their wedding did she say, I, Cynthia, take you, Husband, to be my lawful wedded husband, and did she for the rest of her life go to the foot of their stairs and call out Husband when she wanted him. And did he, Husband –

All very fascinating, Dara said.

No, wait, Femi said. This is what the point is. Did he, I'm certain that he did, spend the whole of his life thinking about what it would be like to be a good husband, be a good capital letters Husband. Because maybe he did and maybe I should have done, I'm a good husband, but I don't know.

You don't know what.

If I was a good husband what was Rupert Fitchwell necessary for and why is she, the mother of my son, why is she dressing still like that, putting on her clothes hoping that the doorbell's going to ring and there will be Rupert Fitchwell.

You're drunk.

He was somehow naked, lying back on the neat duvet cover. His belly had swollen in the last year, his arms no thicker than they had been. His dick and balls lolled on his thigh. Useless, she allowed herself to think.

Who were those people you hated, she said.

What people.

When you came in from your walk with William, she said. You said you hated some people, you wouldn't care if they were removed from the face of the earth. Who were you talking about.

Whom.

Whom then.

You don't care.

All the same I'm asking.

If you don't know the people I'm talking about, you should be thankful, Femi said. I'm going to sleep. It's late. I said it's late. It's late.

I am in the chair in one room. He is in bed in one room. The light is dark in the street. It is half past three but it is not night.

I feel bad, I say.

Or I might say. I am on my own in the room. He is on his own in that room. Time goes by.

I might die, I say. I do not say. I might have said it but I did not.

It is fine that I might die. I do not mind. Now it is dark.

Do you think the plants are all right, I say. He does not hear me speak.

I get up. I feel stiff. I have been in the chair for some time. I cannot say how long. I walk out of the room. I go to where he is, in bed. He looks at me.

What did you say, he says.

You don't look good, I say.

I know, he says. But not as bad as two days back.

Time passes.

Is that what you said, he says.

I don't know, I say.

Then I think.

Do you think the plants are all right, I say.

Is that what you said, he says.

I think.

What plants, he says.

Out the back, the plants, I say.

There is no sound. He has closed his eyes. There is sleep there. I do not say that I might die.

My phone makes a sound. I look. It is some news. I touch the screen and I read.

The curiously affectless quality of sentences like these, I read.

Then I look at the start. It has my name on it. I wrote this and I read a book first and I wrote about it. It was some time back I wrote this.

The curiously affectless quality of sentences like these, I read again.

I go out of the room. I go to the back door. Now I am short of breath. The air in my lungs makes a noise and I feel faint. I look out. I do not want to go out.

There are black bags on the ground there. They have food in them, old food. I see a thing move and it is not a mouse. When I see a thing move it might be a cat, a squirrel, a bird, a mouse, but it is not a mouse. It is a rat, a big rat. I have not seen a rat before in our house or in the back space of our house. The door is there and I am here and the rat is there. It is closed, the door, but it is just there, the rat, I mean. It looks up at me, a big brown rat, and fat, and it walks away. There is no rush and it will be back. It might be the end of the world, when the rats come out to walk in the sun and hunt, and I do not mind.

Oh, no, I think, but it was not fear I felt or not much. There is a rat there. Things have got bad so now there is a rat there.

These days I can voice a bad thing, like there is a rat there and is it the end of the world, or I can say I think I might die now and it does not make me feel much. It is just a fact, it is there and I am here. I am ill and hot and I cannot breathe. I should test that. Test the air that I can, test how much I can. Oxygen: that is the thing. The rat out there I have seen, that is all right and that can wait, I think.

Where is the thing, I say. He is in bed and I am in the same room.

The thing I mean, I say.

Oximeter, I say.

There, he says.

I felt faint, I say.

I put the thing on my finger, the fourth. The ping goes.

What does it say, he says.

It says I say. I look. Eighty-six, I say.

What should it be, he says.

My head hurts, I say. I saw a rat.

A rat, he says.

It says eighty-six on this thing, I say. Eighty-three, I mean.

Ask Mark, he says. But then he picks up his phone and he sends a text. Time passes. I sit on the bed.

A text comes back. I hear the ping.

He says call them, he says. He says call them now.

Call who, I say.

Them, them, them, he says. The people, the doctors, the ones who come out, in their, the, the, the, the ambulance, the ambulance. Can you call? He says you have to call, call them.

His voice hurts him and he stops. His eyes shut. I feel ill too. I look for my phone and it is in my hand. The number to call comes to me and I call it.

Dara thought that love could be precisely measured. Otherwise, how would you know whether you loved somebody more than another? Or whether your love was really as vast and vegetable as it seemed to you, compared with the love other people had for strangers? For her it could be compared to other vast and once imponderable forces, like wind or heat. There was a scale of the ferocity of different chilli peppers, called the Scoville: why not a scale of love? She had a tidy mind, Dara, and she would welcome some objective demonstration of just how much more she loved, for instance, William, than …

She paused in her thoughts, lying there in bed in the dark, staring in the direction of the ceiling.

How much more she loved William than she loved Femi. For instance.

She did not quite know what she would do with the measurement, once tabulated and verified. But she knew that the measurement would be based on one thing, the stories of loss and deprivation you told yourself. The measure of love was the force a narrative held, taking the thing you loved away from you, the story that had never happened and never would, but which the love in your brain constructed and presented to you, complete.

There was the story that Dara told herself, almost every day, and it was a measure of the love she had for her son that there was no dismissing it. Once it had been strangers in her story, taking William away: a kidnapper, lifting her baby from the Silver Cross pushchair while her attention was elsewhere (it was only seconds, and he was under a stranger's overcoat). Or a stranger showing William a picture of some puppy dogs in the park, no, the promise of chocolate and cake, no, that would not tempt her abstemious and delicate son, and soon the stranger in Dara's head had learnt the most important thing about William somehow and had approached him with a beautiful copy of *The Wizard of Oz* with illustrations, the promise that at his house there were so many beautiful books, ones you would never find in a bookshop or a library, and William's eyes growing large and his little steps following, entranced, in the stranger's path to a house, which, in the event, had only ever had one book in it, the beautiful copy of *The Wizard of Oz*. Preserved and kept carefully, in order to serve its one purpose, and never read.

It had always been the story of a stranger taking her William away that had provided a measure of her love for him. When she told these stories to herself, in terror, the world became like the surface of the sea, glistening and vast, and swallowing her love without any sign, any track to follow. But now that had changed. They were no longer strangers taking him away, in her head. Every day now, when Femi said he would go out with William for a walk and the two of them left the house, the door shut behind them and the story she would rather not tell began. It was a sign of everything human in her, the way that her imagination went out and made something so horrible that had never happened and never would happen. She had to do it and she wished it was not necessary.

The door would shut behind Femi and William. They would turn right, as if going to Battersea Park. William would be chattering about his day, about the book he had read that day. He had read so much, considering how old he was; in Dara's story, he would never have the chance to read all the books he would want to. Femi was holding William's hand quite firmly. They walked quickly. A neighbour was approaching them. Femi crossed the road to avoid her. They reached the Queenstown Road. William was no longer talking. He looked big-eyed, afraid; he knew something was wrong. He could not evade what was coming. Soon they had reached the gate to

Battersea Park, but did not go in. They continued on the pavement outside the park, running along the railings, until they reached the bridge. It was white-painted, iron, elaborate. It was the way that you walked to get to Chelsea. Today William and Femi would not get to Chelsea. Femi walked William forcibly to the middle of the bridge, his hand held tightly. Then an end came to the story. He awkwardly manoeuvred himself onto the parapet of the bridge, dragging William with him. He would not let his grip falter for a moment. He jumped; William screaming; the fall through air, the slap and blunder of the river closing over the two of them. All the time Dara waiting at home. She might be cooking them dinner. Perhaps a shepherd's pie. William gone. The story went out into a possible future, painting the spaces and places it might inhabit. It would not go away, and that was the story Dara told herself. She lay in her bed, staring upwards where the ceiling must be, and listened to the heavy breathing of her husband, getting near to sleep, or perhaps just pretending to. William was only a room away, and that was the reality. Tomorrow there would be another moment to face, when he departed the house with his father.

And the novel is not just the story you make up and tell, but the story that your people have told themselves, the ones they want to hear and the ones that are the last thing they want to hear. The ones they read and listen to as well. They reach out. They follow a story. They are human.

William liked to read in bed. He liked reading at all times, but especially he liked reading in bed. Tonight he was reading a story – it was babyish, but he liked it – in *The Pink Fairy Book*. He only read it when he was certain he would not be observed: the judgement of the world on William reading *The Pink Fairy Book* would be swift and final. His bedroom bookshelves were deep, and he kept the twelve *Fairy Books* in a secondary row, behind the front books whose spines could be seen.

One Christmas long ago – it was like the beginning of one of the *Fairy Books'* tales – one of his presents had been George. He was a toy soldier with a scar on his face, eight inches high. His father had talked to him about George more earnestly than a Christmas present generally merited, fixing his eyes on George as a dog would; he had wondered why at the time. Now he thought that his father had decided that he, William, should be the sort of boy to play with soldier toys. Did you say 'play with'? 'Devise adventures for', perhaps would be a more acceptable turn of phrase. At the end of the earnest conversation William had told his father and his mother, who had not been saying anything, that he was going to call his soldier toy George. George was a better order of human being, and pink. His mother had smiled; his father had looked serious.

Outside their house, the cherry tree was in blossom, a burst like a burst of spray foaming up once a rock had fallen into water, a flurry of white, like a whirling girl doing the can-can in her lace petticoats. He liked to think of it still going on, even though it was in the dark and outside. He had drawn his father's attention to it. It had made the peace, after his father had hit him. That had not happened before, not in the street.

Sometimes you kept things to yourself, and one of those turned out to be George. He shouldn't have told that Olu that George had a name, for instance. That Olu, he would never be friends with him if they went to the same school. He had come round with his parents that time from Bromley, where they lived. He didn't know how his parents knew Olu's parents, but they had come round and the two of them had been sent upstairs to play quietly. Olu's sister was too little. She stayed downstairs with the grown-ups. Olu did not read books; he went round William's room in silence, picking things up and putting them down again. He was keen on football; he was in the under-11s first team in Bromley. When he got to the bookcase he put out an index finger and poked a book, another, then a third. William might have been watching an animal that could not be expected to know what a book was for.

Ba, ba, ba, ba, ba, ba, ba, Olu said, in time with his finger's poking. You read all these books, then?

No, William said. He was aware he was standing nervously in his own room, his right arm hooked behind his back, holding his elbow. Not all of them.

What's the point of books, sitting in a chair like an old lady, yeah, Olu said. This is boring. You got Killer Baby 5?

Is that a book?

Olu hurled himself onto William's bed, clutching his sides in a version of merriment, chuckling and roaring.

He says is Killer Baby 5 a book. Yeah, yeah, that's a book all right, get it from Waterstown, nice Christmas present from your aunty. Killer Baby 5, not heard of Killer Baby 5? It's the best. This baby got to go round killing the old ladies, you earn your weapons, I'm up to nuclear cannon, takes me six months. See one, aim, fire, blam, kill, next old woman. It's the best. Where's your Xbox.

Have you got this, William said. One of these.

He picked up George the regal toy soldier from the top of the chest of drawers. It might be the only thing in William's room that could appeal to someone like Olu.

Oh, yeah, Action Man, Olu said. I had one of them when I was like a baby. You a fan of Action Man, hold him dear to your heart, then? Can have a battle, kill that little teddy over there, a nice interrogation, torture, shoot them, I like your way of thinking.

He's called George, William said.

Who's called George.

The soldier.

He's not called George. How is he called George? That's Action Man. Action Man doesn't have a name, he's like Action Man, what is this, *Toy Story*.

But George did have a name. His name was George. He had to have a name because it was George William told stories to. George listened, his jaw set and his little scar very evident. (One day he would talk back, tell the story of how that scar came about.) He was Action Man in the shop and to people like Olu, but to William he was not to be replaced, and it was George who listened. Tonight he would listen to the best story from *The Pink Fairy Book*, the one about the princess in the chest.

Do you know the story about the princess in the chest, William said to George. But George either did not or was being polite.

Well, there was a king once whose queen never had a child. And he loved her but a king needs a son or daughter. And the king said to the queen, I am going away, and I will stay away for a year, a whole year. When I come back you must have had a baby, or I will execute you with a large axe and marry someone better. And the next day he rode off. Where he went must be a story for another day. The queen wept bitterly, alone in her chamber, but then there was a knock on her door, and it was a small man with a strange sort of red pointed cap on and green pointed shoes, and he said, I can give you a baby of your own, which will be born on the day the king returns, and she will be as beautiful as the day, and as white as yogurt, and as clever as Charlotte Brontë. But the king must not see her and you must not see her once she is born. She must stay alone in a room in the castle and never see her parents until the day of her fourteenth birthday, or she will die. And the queen said …

George fixed him with his unwavering glare; William went on, carefully not forgetting any step in the story, considering and then adding what details he thought might serve. He loved the story; the princess seeming to die; the knight volunteering for the vigil in the church; the monster that howled around him and the steps of his safety. He loved the resurrection of the dead at the end. Most of all he loved that nobody was punished, neither the wicked dwarf nor the king, who seemed to William to be wicked in his own way, nor the howling monster. It seemed just right to William. He went on, telling a story, patient and precise as a mapmaker, getting nothing wrong and leaving nothing out. As he carried on, the unpurged terrors of the day receded and *what happened next* rose up, like a thick velvet curtain, muffling and blood-red, between him and his father next door in bed. Today his father had told William to shut up while they were on their walk, and when William had started talking again, his father had hit him. The princess, or what was left of her, leapt out of her trunk in search of blood. His father faded and shrank. Soon William would finish, George would be on the bedside table, and sleep would come. Night-time was the time to tell yourself a story.

I call them. I shut my eyes. I lie down. He is there too, my man. The door goes. I get up then I have to sit down. They are here, the men.

What seems to be the trouble, one of the men says.

He is large. I think I might have seen him before but I do not know.

I have COVID, I say.

His oxygen levels are very low, my husband says. He seems quite confused.

I feel, I say, but I am not quite sure.

The other man is large too. He puts the thing on my finger, the thing that tests can you breathe. He asks me if I can count from ten back to one. I count. I get it right, I think.

It's low, one of the men says. We'll take him into hospital. Do you have everything you need?

Yes, my husband says. I've packed you a bag, he says, and there it is.

I want to cry. He is so ill too. He packed my bag.

Can we go to St Thomas', I say. They know me there, I've been there before.

We have to take you to the nearest hospital, the man says. That's in Chelsea. We'll be putting the lights on, the siren, we need to get you there. Are you all right to walk?

Both the men have masks on, I see, and they have blue gloves on, blue plastic gloves like the ones the butcher kept in a box outside his shop for his customers to put on, all through this last year.

Are you butchers, I say. I want to chat, to be cheerful. They say nothing.

Let's get you going, one says.

I just want to, I say, and I look at my husband. He never cries but I am crying now and when I go with the men I am crying some more. When I look back and he is there in the door and the van, the ambulance, is there in front with its light on.

And now I am out of the moment I am in. I can see the story that might be before me. I am out of thinking only about me. There are all those other people who said goodbye like this. In my thoughts are other people, people I don't know, people I imagine who perhaps never existed, and I can see who they are and what they went through. This is the first time for days this has happened.

I won't be long, I say. I'll be back soon.

And there were people who said that this year, to their husbands, also going into hospital. To be checked out. And they stayed there. They never saw them again. And those other people. Those who said goodbye, I'll see you soon, to people who were heading off on a journey. A wave, a turn, going back inside, and the person they had said *soon* to never returned. People who said, *I'll see you there*, and for ever afterwards had to remember, that was the last thing they ever said, the last words they ever exchanged. I meant to say something that would mean something, something that showed what I felt, something that was only what I felt and what would reflect what he felt, too. But it was no good. I was in a world of monosyllables and I said what a million people said as the last thing they would ever say to the man they loved, *I'll see you soon, don't fret*.

The truth is that when you are reduced to the warm hard core of yourself one thing remains. Reduced by events. You have no control. And what is left of you is love. I was walked the few steps from front door to ambulance and I only thought one thing, How would he manage when I was not there, Would he eat. Would he sleep. Would he get better, or would he grow ill too, as ill as I was. I wanted him to be safe and I could do nothing about him. I knew above all things that moment when you wake, perhaps on a warm Saturday morning, the daylight beginning to show at the edge of the bedroom curtains, a beautiful, beautiful day. You are awake but your husband is still asleep; you curve yourself about him, and both of you are soon asleep again, warm and pyjama'd, with nothing to do but be there with each other. That was what I thought as I said goodbye. Then I was in the ambulance and I cried and cried, left with nothing but what I felt, the hard warm irreduceable kernel of love.

I reached, too, for the word I could remember, a word of real terror, as the man in the ambulance, a stranger, held my hand. I wanted to explain why I had said to him *Are you butchers* but now I was not sure if I had said that or why. The word that came to me was *intubation*. It came to me with a sinister hush, not contained in a sentence. The world fell quiet and this word was spoken. I wondered why it had come to me with such force. *Intubation*. I wondered what it meant. The noise of wail and the light outside, the circling light on the ambulance, went on. We were moving, fast. I fell back into darkness. I slept.

In the hard dark centre of the night, the long silences Femi had endured were broken. Their bedroom was at the front of the house. Femi remembered that once you walked down streets like this, and every upper window in every house was darkened by the back of a dressing-table. Their room was not like that; Dara had no dressing-table, but prepared herself in the bathroom and from the top of the chest of drawers, where brushes, mascara, lipstick lived. One wall was sealed in by fitted bedroom furniture, sliding doors in pale oak around a central long mirror. There were small bedside cabinets to either side of the bed; a shoe rack under the window; a small button-back armless chair upholstered in dark green velvet, and the walls painted a heavy, sombre purplish-brown.

Now there was a sound and a loud light in the street. It was a circling orange blare that cut through the crack between the heavy midnight-blue curtains. Dara slept. Her position was one that no person could hold for long awake. Her arm was flung up, her elbow cornering and framing her face. He glanced at her. His head was thumping and his eyes were sore. It was a stupid position she had found herself in. Even in her unconscious state Femi could feel contempt for her. His tongue was thickly coated; there was a hot throb in his neck. He concentrated on it. In the street there was a fierce orange light and a sudden quick crackle of a voice speaking, amplified, an electronic burst of incomprehensible words. It was an ambulance. It was probably three or four or five houses away. He didn't know those people. He wouldn't recognize them if he passed them. He lay there. Quickly a scenario came to him. In it he got up, put on his white towelling dressing-gown, went downstairs, opened the front door and was in the street –

What's this row, maybe-Femi would say.

We're just doing our job, the paramedic in his green uniform said.

It's four in the morning, maybe-Femi would say. He looked, the real Femi, and it was indeed four. He was confirmed.

This gentleman is very ill, the maybe-paramedic said, pointing down. A white man on a stretcher was foaming at the mouth, was flailing around.

My husband, my husband, a maybe-wife said, a white woman. Please help me, she said.

How can I help you, maybe-Femi said. Be reasonable, madam.

And then she would go on to explain that she had three children and nobody to look after them and could he not as a neighbour perhaps let them sleep at his house for the next few nights, just a very few nights, because she had to –

But maybe-Femi had the answer to that, and it was certainly true that the neighbour had never acknowledged him until now, when the Black man could it seemed be useful to her. That was it, and it was too late by far for her to begin to acknowledge and to make friendly gestures in the direction of the existence of maybe-Femi, or maybe real-Femi. Femi lay there, his head pounding, his mouth thick, and his lips moved silently. He was putting her in her place, this imagined woman, but it would do, with many fluently made points of racism and social duty, of obligations undertaken and social trust earned.

He went on, maybe-Femi, with a fluency that was almost like delight. In a few moments he finished. He was almost trembling with the energy of what he had had to say.

Outside, the real circling orange light had continued. Now a door was slammed; a noise started, the furious and yet bedraggled sound of a siren at close quarters. The neighbour in the back of the ambulance was being taken at full speed. Now would have been the moment for the maybe-neighbour to collapse, to be put right, to accept her humble place after she had been crushed by maybe-Femi's contempt. But she did not. She had disappeared. Femi had made his maybe-points crushingly, cogently, like a machine for squaring things off and despatching them for ever, and once the points had been made, he was left standing there. He had one thing left to observe, there in his triumph.

None of this happened.

He brought that knowledge to mind.

As if a pair of heavy curtains had opened, and another, and a third set behind, and finally the significant object was revealed with a terrible clarity. He understood exactly what he had done, and in a moment he understood his poor self-created life as a simple fact. He had invented a scenario in which people were horrible and evil. He had created a triumph for himself, crushing enemies under his tread. But none of it had happened. People in reality were good and patient. They had done and would do nothing wrong. The only one in his head who was not good and patient, who would do wrong in the world, was him.

He had done all of this to himself.

The brief blare of siren took place outside in the street. The vehicle left. It did not disturb Dara, who slept on. Presently a new noise began, a white noise of precipitation. It was rain. At first it was a light hiss; as it continued, it grew heavier, with a true weight of weather in it, drumming on surface and vessel, on vehicle and roof. It was above and outside and beneath and it would not stop. The waters fell from the heavens to the earth. Nobody but Femi was alive and awake to hear it. Only Femi heard the full power of it, the water that had been swept up from the seas to hover over the land in great black clouds, to break at last and to bring the saltless masses of the ocean down over England, over London, over this suburb, this corner, this street, this house, this head. He listened and then he merely heard.

The noise stops and the movement stops. The door is opened into a world of rain. There are two men in masks there. They ask if I can walk. I say yes. But I get out of the ambulance and I have to hold on. They get a chair for me.

Then I am in a room. There are things all round me in this room, all working, with lights and sounds. I could guess what some of them do. But I do not know and I do not know what the names of these things are.

We're going to put you on oxygen, a man says.

I say nothing.

In a while I am in the chair and a mask is on my face. I can hear its sibilance.

Time goes by.

A man comes in who I have not seen. He places a pair of hard blocks of stuff on my chest and he says, This is to do an X-ray in bed, where I am. This is the first time I have heard of this. I thought you had to go to an X-ray room and that the machines that did the X-ray were big and fixed and could not move. But it works.

There is oxygen going into me. I feel so dizzy still.

This is a room I have not been in before. It smells just as my house has smelt in the last week or two weeks. It smells of the oven that has not been cleaned. I need to clean the oven but how is that smell here when the oven is at home.

What is wrong with me.

I know what is wrong with me. It is a long time since I paid any attention to someone else. I could not tell you at the moment whether I have been looked after by two people or by twelve. They come into this room and I do not recognize or remember them.

I have been here for I don't know how long.

The man who comes into the room next is sheltered by a big plastic mask like the others. His hands are covered with blue transparent gloves. Under the gloves he wears a wedding ring. I am wearing a wedding ring too. And this forms a bond between us but not the same bond that is formed by my wearing one wedding ring and my husband wearing another wedding ring. His ring is made of white gold and my ring is made of yellow gold. This thought seems profound to me. I want to share it with the man.

I wonder where the other half of his wedding-ring-wearing pair is. If it is a man who wears the other ring, or a woman. He or she might be black, as this man is, or white, or Asian, like the man I am married to, or another ethnicity. I wonder if he or she is a doctor, or another profession, or if he or she stays at home and looks after the children.

The man in the room with the wedding ring under his blue plastic gloves is steady and careful. His presence is warm and he looks at me in a kind, human way. He is not scared. I can see the woman he is married to, calm and clever, and his children, three daughters, also clever and kind, one good at sports, at hockey, another a good player of the clarinet. The thoughts are frail; they fade quickly, and they never quite had faces I could believe in.

The oxygen goes into me. The room slows and calms. I am thinking about the family of a man I have never met before, who has so far said nothing. It seems to me that I have not wondered about another human being for weeks. I have been shut in my own mind, my own circumstances. I could not read a novel because other people were out there, beyond the walls of my illness. I could not think of them. I had become someone who never read novels, who talked about themselves. I might have been the Stalinist across the road.

The doctor's big luminous face is close to mine. It is separated from me by a thick transparent plastic screen. I want to tell him all these things now. But it is hard for me to turn the thoughts into sense, and in a moment he starts to talk, to explain things to me. His voice is deep and slow. Once he has said some things he checks that I have taken it in. I nod. I will be fine. I will stay here for a while. But I will get well. I will get well.

His wife waits for him.

His girls too.

I hope that the shield, the mask, the gloves, the protection, all that is enough. I hope with everything I have to hope that his family, his wife and daughters, greet a sanitized and infection-free father at the end of his shift. I have invented these people. I want them to stay well. I want this illness with its confusions and its vertigo and its sweats at night to stop with me. I want to go home. I want to get well.

The night possessed only one noise, the sound of water plummeting from the heavens to the earth. Precipitation. It was only Femi who could not sleep. He lay for an hour with the din outside for company. The woman who was his wife was on her side, facing away from him. The Book of Exodus came to him, and Moses. You will see my back parts; but my face shall not be seen. He had won a prize for Bible knowledge when he was a boy. Some of it still came to him. There were days when God reminded you that his face could not be seen. He would turn his back. The back of the person who could have saved you was turned to you, too. Her face was away from him, and it would never be turned to him again. It looked away, and it was engrossed by Mr Rupert Fitchwell. What was left for Femi was the construction of dialogues that had never taken place and never would, dialogues where he triumphed over the world – not even that, but a world in which he had a place and a value. He had to imagine that, because it would not take place otherwise.

The rains roared. The object that was his life, revealed to him by the parting of those curtains in the head: he could take that in his hand and do what he would with it. There was no reason for him not to do what he had often thought of doing. The means of doing it had often gone through his mind – a knife from the kitchen, a stretch of rope, a bottle of pills, even, extravagantly, the acquisition of a gun from somewhere. Now it was clear to him that the act must be silent. He did not want to wake his wife or his son by crying out, or by his heels drumming on the wall, and this was not consideration, he recognized, but by a simple fear that they might prevent the conclusion. He walked downstairs barefoot. Underfoot there was the carpet they had chosen together, the colour she had insisted on. In the dark, just then, he could not remember what colour it was. He walked up and down it thirty times a day, as well. All at once the matter was childishly simple. He went in the dark to the kitchen drawer where such things were kept. He got out three plastic bags and, scrabbling around a little, some rubber bands. They felt strong enough. He almost congratulated himself on his ingenuity, going into the sitting room and shutting the door behind him.

The door opened in front of me. Between me and it was rain, a cataract. The framed yellowish light of my hallway was like an aubade. I was home. My husband stood in the framed doorway in his plump-shouldered purple dressing-gown, having seen the ambulance that had brought me home.

Soon I would be better. I would no longer be myself, with my gaze fixed on my own self alone. The people around me would grow interesting again, whether they were people I spent every day with, like my beautiful and clever husband, full of the wonders of a personality to be explored over the course of years, or a man I glimpsed once in the street, his carriage, clothing, expression, gestures evoking a whole life. The transcript of the unknown would come back, to the point of creating the impossible.

A sentence from a novel: *Many years later, as he faced the firing squad, Colonel Aureliano Buendia was to remember that distant afternoon when his father took him to see the ice.* The novel and the art it embodied, both in those who wrote them and those who read them, was an interlacing of the truth and the invented. What happened passed before the eyes, and it was drab, monosyllabic, solipsistic, inadequate once transcribed; what might have happened stretched out limitlessly, rooted in and always returning to what had been seen.

My husband took the bag he had packed from the paramedic. Both of them stretched out to do this, keeping their distance. Then he put his arms around me. I was wet. He did not cry, as a matter of practice. I was the great weeper in the marriage, at moments of tiredness, at films, at sights in the garden or at the breaking of a tea bowl. I felt his warmth against mine and I thought how he must have spent these last hours, waiting. The paramedic who had brought me and my bag to my front door muttered something awkward, from the safe distance he was observing. He went back to the ambulance. We went inside and shut the door. My husband brought me a towel and tea and we sat side by side, on the sofa. It was nearly five in the morning. Soon the dawn would come.

How was it, he said.

They were, I said. I don't know. Efficient, perhaps. I can't imagine how they carry on.

And they have to put up with people applauding them all the time, he said.

That's the worst of it, I said. But listen. This very strange thing happened.

I started to talk; a tall story. After a while my husband said, Oh, come on. I carried on. His face was alight with disbelieving amusement. The story I had to tell him lasted another half an hour, and the only truth it had in it was the way a nurse had come into the room backwards. She was broad-hipped in her blue nylon uniform and, when she turned, had a saucy snub nose. Coming in backwards, she had knocked a paper cup full of water off the table, and had said with real feeling, Oh, for fuck's sake. She had apologized; that had been the end of it. My story of what might have happened after that went on. It drew on what I had seen; it went into what the nurse might have felt, knowing that the person who was among those applauded every Thursday at six was not a person who would ever say *for fuck's sake* in front of a patient. It was a good story. I would work on it. It was not true. In the morning I thought I might take it easy; read a novel. One day I might feel like writing some of this down.

William walked down the stairs. He was barefoot and careful as he trod. All the doors in the house were shut. They normally stood open. There was no reason to shut them, in normal circumstances. But now his mother had gone round shutting them. He knew that something considerable had happened; he knew that he would remember this morning's waking for the rest of his life, and refer to it often, in conversation with new friends, strangers, colleagues. All that would come in time, and carefully, left foot, right foot, he walked down the staircase. His mother was in the kitchen, on her phone. It sounded as if she was talking to somebody official from the commanding tone of her voice. William made a mental note of that. He would not have known what a woman sounds like after discovering the body of her husband. He might have guessed that she would scream, and wail, and tear her hair, or at the very least cry. It was interesting that a woman did not, but got through the practical steps with a firm, serious voice, as if addressing a classroom.

The voice in the kitchen broke off and, with a touch more urgency, called to him.

Come here, his mother's voice said, raised. Don't go in there. Don't go in the sitting room, I mean.

William paused. He regretted what his mother had said. He would have been interested to see his father's dead body. It would have been interesting, too, to know what it felt like to see that, the specific surge of emotion. Would he cry? Or would he faint at the horrible sight, crying all the time, Father, my father? It would be worth knowing, and learning the truth of the matter from life, and not what had been written many times before. He would not disobey his mother and go into the room with the now strangely closed door, however. He was satisfied to learn that she stayed where she was, in the kitchen, instead of coming out to seize him. He wondered why. Perhaps she would not want to see the door that she had closed. That was also a possibility.

William took the three steps forward that led him to the front door. Soon an ambulance would come, or perhaps just a doctor in a car. He did not know which it would be. They would enter a house where a dead body was, and they would carry themselves in particular ways. But he did not need to know that. He knew exactly what their stance and carriage would be.

William, the voice said from behind him. He opened the door. He knew what would be there and he stepped forward into it. The waters lapped about his ankles, soaking the bottom cuff of his blue pyjamas with the black floral pattern. The waters stretched in front of him; they were green, and brown, and here and there a swipe of floating oil on the surface shimmered with the blue of a peacock's tail. All above the sky was clear and cold, and cerulean; William knew the exact word for its colour.

It must have been raining all night, and where the street had been was now a lake. The water was cold, but not unpleasant. The rains had passed, and the sky was cloudless. He shut the door behind him on the house with the dead father in it, and waded forward. The row of houses opposite his front door had been done away with, and the street beyond that. In the waters, calm and smooth and the colour of dust, only some buildings and structures remained. The church on the place where the Queenstown Road had been still stood, three hundred yards away, apparently floating in water. A pillarbox made a point in the sheet of water further away, like a single exclamation mark on a blank page. The houses were gone, and the shops too; most human habitation, and most humans with them. If William turned, his right foot dragging the cold weight of water with it, like a vast cloak, he would see that the house he had come from had now been abolished too. He was alone in the cold weight of water, an expanse that pressed forward in all directions to the horizon. He would not know what that expanse of water contained unless he went forward. It was a vivid clean blue-lit morning, cold and open; he waded in a new world of water with its few monuments occasional and mean-ingless. Cerulean; moss-green; gamboge; the dull brown of earth in woodland underneath everything.

Trees rose from the flat, shining lake-expanse. The only sounds were those of birds, going from one red-varnished cherry-tree branch to another, sitting in the high lime-green frilled twigs of the ginkgo. They were quite satisfied with this new world; they did not need to tread on the ground that had been lost. And as if to confirm it, a family of ducks, swimming bumptiously past him, the mother brown, the father with a radiant blue-green head and neck, like the slicks of petrol on the surface of the water. Behind them a small squadron of ducklings swam, buffeting each other and busily progressing in a mob. William took a step forward. They flurried away. It did not matter. Under the surface of the water, a languid curl of muscle. A large carp, coming to William, had investigated him and was turning away. It was big enough to eat a duckling, but did not.

The trees marked the places where the streets had been. In the absence of the houses, they marked out a double line of progression, a surprisingly stately avenue rising from the waters. It occurred to William that some of the land formed small hills, or had done until now. It might have been expected that some of these small hills might rise from the flat expanse of the water to form islands. But that had not happened. Instead, there was a lake, or an inland sea, stretching as far as could be surveyed. In one direction, a large clump of trees in the water showed where the common had been; in the other, quite far away but visible, the shining gates of the park, and behind them, dense copses and woodland. He took a step forward in an irresolute way. In the air hung what might have been an echo of the woman's call: William, William, William. It echoed and rang, the shadow of a sound that had never, in this world, sounded. The water was heavy about his legs; he walked forward. Underneath his bare feet he could feel the gritty texture of what had once been pavement. He decided to turn right, and to go to Battersea Park.

Beyond that was the River. He wanted to see what had happened to it.

He struggled on. The water was cold and opaque. It pulled and swished about his knees. It had grown deeper, somehow. He wondered if he would ever get to Battersea Park, or if the swelling waters would rise up to such a height, or such a depth, that he would have to swim to get there. He looked again, and the gates of the park might be what he could see: a flash of gold in the light of the sun. Or that might be the pillars of the bridge beyond; or it might be the flash of the sun on the waters. He could swim, he supposed, but he would reach no landmark to haul himself out on, nothing but the possibility of a tree in whose uppermost branches he could perch, like one of the savage swift neon-green parakeets, whose shrieks were rending the air about him. It might be that he would have to turn around, to go back to the house he had left. But the house he had left was gone, erased and with nothing but the flat green-grey shining waters in its place. There was no returning home today, and only onwards into deepening waters. It was not sinister or threatening, that prospect of deepening waters. William would find a passage across or through them some-how, he was sure of that. He did not see how, exactly, but the solution would come to him in time.

The trees stood singly for the most part, isolated in the water. William wondered if it would be good for trees to sit in standing water like mangroves. (Even now, with his father dead and everything expended for no purpose, he was pleased with himself for knowing what mangroves were.) He stopped his steady progress through the heaviest of the elements, the

moving and unmoving and whole and united body of water
that stretched in all directions. It must stretch as far as the sea,
obliterating the path of the River and the shape of the estuary.
He dipped his finger into the flood, and first sniffed, then
tasted it. He knew that cholera and worse could be carried by
standing waters in a flood, the sewers of the city broken and
pouring out. Still he tentatively licked his wet finger. There
was, surely, some salt in it as well as river water; the flood was
brackish. Another word he was pleased with himself for knowing. He felt like setting it down. But in this world, so far, there
was no paper, no means of keeping paper dry if it existed, and
no way of preserving it from the obliterations of the flood.
Still, he wanted to write the word *brackish* down as something
he had observed and understood and knew how to name.

If he turned, away from the sun which was still hanging in
the east, he could see two thick heavy trees standing close to
each other, their upper branches and foliage intimately
involved. They were densely foliaged, dark and glossy, like
houseplants rather than outside trees. Their shapes, reflected,
shimmered in the still water that came three feet up their
dark trunks. About them, fat yellow fruit bobbed in the
waters like lost beach balls. William waded towards the trees.
Presently he came close, and found himself among the floating fruit. He picked one from the grey water, dripping, and
tore its thick skin. Inside, the flesh was pink, segmented,
juicy; he raised it to his face and smelt the sour fragrance
within the all-enveloping brackish, ferny, salt-edged smell.
There was something that was not grapefruit. And then a
woman was there; her thin linen skirt tucked up into her
knickers, wading to greet him, picking the fruit from the
water as she came.

I've seen you, she said. She was bright-faced, her hands big,
her teeth long and white, but old, her hair tied up in a stretch

of cloth. I've seen you before, looking at the trees! You like trees?

William said he did.

I like them too, the woman said. I am a person who likes the trees, and grows them. Do you know what these trees are? They are called pomeloes. And one day I succeeded in growing them here, in this country, and not in the country that I am born in, which is Grenada. My name is Marianne. Take as many as you like. Put them in the boat.

I'm William. I don't have a boat, William said.

You don't have a boat! And all this water we have to deal with, these days! Some days it is fire, some days earth, and some days water.

And every day there is air, William said. Or we would die.

Yes, that's so, Marianne said, her face creasing up with joyous, silent laughter. I see you know your onions, William.

Still, William said, I don't seem to have a boat.

I was not suggesting as a matter of fact that you have a boat, Marianne said. I am teasing you, as you will understand if you hang around here much longer. What I am suggesting is that you put the pomeloes in this boat, my boat, and then if you would like to borrow the boat, take it and bring it back when you are done.

William looked, and indeed, that was correct, that round the middle trunk of the nearer of the two trees there floated an orange inflatable dinghy, tied securely. He knew those inflatable dinghies, so leathery and so inflated that their surface seemed hard, that a flick of a fingernail would make a deep hollow sound. This dinghy was inflated as fully as it would go. He had not noticed it before, but now he thought Marianne had made a good suggestion, that he could borrow it and take it where he wanted to go. For many weeks he had wanted to go beyond the street they lived in, with the few trees, the few lives within it. He had wanted, sometimes quite passionately, to go to Battersea Park. There, behind the gates that were glittering in the sun half a mile away, glittering and waist deep in the tranquil lake the rains had made, was a world of trees, of floating plants, of swans liberated from their confines that could now swim anywhere. He had been lent a dinghy by Marianne, laden with fruit from her two trees. He, too, could now go anywhere by floating on the surface of the waters. He did not know where he would go after Battersea Park, but the dinghy would take him there. And then when he was done – at whatever point that would be – he could bring it back.